Simple Things You Can Do to Help Prevent Cancer

- Eat a Diet Rich in Beta-Carotene—Choose from a list of foods that are rich in beta-carotene, which can suppress and even reverse some cancers.

- Cook Meats at Lower Temperatures—Try oven-roasting, baking, microwaving, stewing, boiling or poaching, as charred meat contains carcinogens.

- Perform Regular Breast and Skin Self-exams—Follow the simple, step-by-step instructions provided.

- Eat Broccoli—It is a major source of sulforaphane, one of the most powerful anticancer compounds found in foods.

- Boost Your Intake of Dietary Fiber—You'll cut your risk of colon cancer by 50 percent! A high-fiber diet may also reduce your risk of breast and stomach cancers.

- Use Nontoxic Cleaning Products—Disinfectants account for the largest pesticide use in homes.

ALSO BY ROBERTA ALTMAN

Waking Up, Fighting Back:
The Politics of Breast Cancer

The Cancer Dictionary

The Prostate Answer Book

The Complete Book of Home
Environmental Hazards

Every Woman's Handbook for Preventing Cancer

MORE THAN 100 SIMPLE WAYS
TO REDUCE YOUR RISK

Roberta Altman

POCKET BOOKS

New York   London   Toronto   Sydney   Tokyo   Singapore

The author of this book is not a physician and the ideas, procedures, and suggestions in this book are not intended as a substitute for the medical advice of a trained health professional. All matters regarding your health require medical supervision. Consult your physician before adopting the suggestions in this book, as well as about any condition that may require diagnosis or medical attention. The author and publisher disclaim any liability arising directly or indirectly from the use of the book.

An *Original* Publication of POCKET BOOKS

POCKET BOOKS, a division of Simon & Schuster Inc.
1230 Avenue of the Americas, New York, NY 10020

ISBN: 0-671-52280-9

First Pocket Books trade paperback printing October 1996

10   9   8   7   6   5   4   3   2   1

POCKET and colophon are registered trademarks of
Simon & Schuster Inc.

Text design by Stanley S. Drate/Folio Graphics Co. Inc.

Printed in the U.S.A.

To all women, young and old, who have not gotten their fair share of medical attention and care. And to Mom, Melissa and Cheryl Altman, Rochelle Smith, Ruth Premselaar, Judy Berkman, Sandy Levy, Katherine Kelleher, Susan Pringle, Janet Schoene, Hilary Ziff, Tina Mosetis, Beverly Poppell, Nancy Pline, and Midori Fukaishi who have always given me more than my fair share of caring, support, and love.

ℒℴ

Acknowledgments

Much appreciation to the following organizations for making so much material available to me and answering so many (at times frantic) questions: American Institute for Cancer Research; United States Department of Agriculture/Human Nutrition Information Service; Public Citizen/Health Research Group; Indoor Air Quality Information Clearinghouse (IAQ/INFO); American Cancer Society (ACS); Centers for Disease Control and Prevention (CDC); Leukemia Society of America; National Cancer Institute (NCI); National Coalition for Cancer Survivorship (NCCS); Skin Cancer Foundation; U.S. Food and Drug Administration (FDA); TSCA Assistance Information Service; Breast Implant Information Network; National Alliance of Breast Cancer Organizations (NABCO); Center for Science in the Public Interest; United Soybean Hotline; Greenpeace; Women's Environment and Development Organization (WEDO); U.S. Environmental Protection Agency (EPA); Center for Science in the Public Interest; National Coalition for Alternatives to Pesticides (NCAP); Public Citizen; Action on Smoking and Health (ASH); Office on Smoking and Health at CDC.

Thanks also to my editors, Emily Bestler and Amelia Sheldon, and my agent, Janis Vallely, all of whom offered unconditional encouragement and support.

Contents

INTRODUCTION   *1*

I *Your Body*   9

II *Your Home and Workplace*   155

III *Your Environment*   181

THE MOST COMMON CANCERS AFFECTING
   WOMEN IN 1996   205

GLOSSARY   217

ORGANIZATIONS AND RESOURCES   231

COMPREHENSIVE CANCER CENTERS   245

BIBLIOGRAPHY   249

INDEX   253

Introduction

When I discovered a small lump in my breast in 1976, I was very frightened. I knew virtually nothing about breast cancer other than the fact that a lump in the breast could be the disease. My gynecologist told me to relax, that it was nothing, and that I should come back and see her in six months. I was too anxious to take her advice and insisted on having the lump removed. I was thirty-four years old when I heard the words, "I'm sorry, the lump was malignant." I had my breast removed and went on with my life.

But my life was never the same. Any little thing out of the ordinary in my body provoked fear that the cancer had returned. When it did return in 1981, my prognosis was grim. When I asked my oncologist how long I'd be on chemotherapy, he told me for the rest of my life, thinking that I'd be around for about eighteen months. I was terrified. I was also very angry and determined to fight this latest assault on my life. I got as much information as I could find about breast cancer. It fit easily into a large manila envelope. Nowhere could I find information on what caused my breast cancer, what I could have done to prevent it. The dearth of knowledge was astounding, especially when my research showed me how many women in the United States were getting breast cancer and how many were dying.

1

While working on a book on the politics of breast cancer a dozen years later, I realized that there was still very little known about breast cancer—its cause, its prevention, and treatment that worked. Women with symptoms or a diagnosis of breast cancer are always being referred to me by friends. I tell them my story, but I cannot tell them why I got breast cancer when no one else in my family had ever had it or why I am the lucky one who survived. I always want to be able to give them more information. This is a humble attempt.

One cancer that I have for which I do know the cause is skin cancer. As I was growing up, most of my summer days were spent at the beach. We lived in Westchester, New York, with a beach nearby. My father's family lived in Brooklyn, blocks from the Atlantic Ocean. The highlight of my summer was our annual visit to Jones Beach. Being freckled (did I hate that) and fair-skinned, I had many a bad sunburn even though my parents tried to keep me covered and under an umbrella. In those days it was simply not known how harmful, years later, those painful sunburns could be. I now see a dermatologist twice a year. I've had numerous skin cancers removed. Since sun damage to the skin cannot be repaired, my visits to the dermatologist will continue throughout my lifetime. Today we know that hundreds of thousands of skin cancers like my own can be easily avoided by limiting our exposure to the sun.

We now know a lot more about cancer than we did years ago. But there is still a tremendous amount that we don't know about its causes and prevention. In this book I will share the latest information available on various risk factors for different cancers. There are two categories of risk factors: those over which we have no control, such as age and genes, and those that we can do something about, such as diet and cigarette smoking.

A major risk factor over which we, as women, have no control is just being a woman. Women who are working are more likely than men to have low-paying jobs with no medical coverage or a very meager policy, which puts us at a greater risk of not getting the best medical treatment and therefore not surviving cancer. Women who are covered by their husband's insurance are likely to lose it if their husband dies or they get a divorce. A study done by the Older Women's League (OWL) in 1992 reported that only 55 percent of women aged forty to forty-six have health insurance on their jobs, while 72 percent of men in the same age group have coverage at their jobs. In addition, the male medical establishment has put far more resources into research on men's ailments. A recent National Cancer Institute (NCI) study, for example, found that men who shun vegetables and are overweight are at a significantly higher risk for developing esophageal cancer than their normal weight, vegetable-eating counterparts (but where were the women in that study??!). Other studies have looked at electromagnetic field exposure and male breast cancer (yet only 1 percent of all breast cancer cases occur in men!).

Although there are risk factors over which we have no control, being aware of them can make the difference between surviving or succumbing. Knowing about a specific risk factor can enable you to do things to counter its impact to as great an extent as possible. For example, if there is a long history of breast cancer in your family, you may see your doctor and have mammograms more often than is generally recommended or get into a breast surveillance group if one is available.

When I started doing research for this book, I thought I was pretty aware of the risk factors for cancer. I was amazed at the number of other possible risk factors I found of which I had not been aware. I've included all that I've come across, even the ones that are suspect but for which there is little conclusive proof. There have been so many instances of a theory's being pooh-poohed only to find, years later, that it was correct and that having that information and using it could have saved lives.

Obviously, some factors pose a large risk and others pose a much smaller one, but it is combinations of factors, large and small, that may be responsible for the development of many cancers. Therefore, while exposure to a small amount of a carcinogen may not in and of itself cause cancer, when it is combined with exposures to small amounts of other carcinogens, cancer may result. For example, if you smoke and you are also exposed to radon in your home or at work, your risk of getting lung cancer is exponentially increased. The effect of different factors together may be greater than the sum of their effects separately. As more research is done, more and more risk factors are being identified and their roles in the development of cancer are becoming better defined.

Many known and suspected risk factors can be avoided with just a little effort, such as changing the kind of oil you use when you cook or doing a little more exercise every day. Avoiding other risk factors may require a major lifestyle change and commitment; smokers face the greatest challenge. Today it is well-documented that cigarette smoking causes lung cancer, which is usually fatal. It is also well-established that people who don't smoke but are exposed to secondhand smoke created by those who do can also develop and die from lung cancer. Smoking has been linked to many other cancers as well. If you are a smoker and continue to smoke, there is no guarantee that you will develop lung cancer. But you've got a much greater chance of hearing those dreaded words, "the biopsy was positive," than someone who doesn't smoke. If you stop smoking, there is no guarantee that you will not get lung cancer, but your risk will decrease over time. And yes, there are people who do not smoke and do develop lung cancer, but they are the exception, not the rule.

There is another risk that I haven't mentioned yet. That is the risk of dying of cancer once you have been diagnosed with it. Ideally, the best approach is to do everything possible to prevent the onset of cancer in the first place. But that is not always possible. The good news is that it has been well-established that in most cases *the earlier cancer is diagnosed and treated, the better the chance it can be cured.* For that reason, I have provided information in this book on screening and symptoms for some cancers. Using that information gives you the best chance of finding a cancer as early as possible, when there is the best hope of successful treatment.

There are three types of cancer prevention: *primary prevention* to keep cancer from ever occurring (which is obviously the best prevention); *secondary prevention,* which seeks to detect the cancer as early as possible so as to ensure the best chance of survival (an example is the use of mammography); and *tertiary prevention* to reduce the rate of recurrence and disability (the treatment of cancer).

The sole purpose of this book is to make you aware of the various risk factors for cancer and what you can do to avoid and reduce them in your life. Although there are

now many books out on cancer, there is no book specifically for women on how they can reduce their risk of
getting cancer. I have designed this book to be as user-
friendly as possible. It is divided into three parts: the risk
factors in your body, the risk factors in your home and
workplace, and the risk factors in the environment. Each
part is arranged alphabetically, and when there is more
than one name for a particular risk factor, there will be
one major entry and the other names will be cross-
referenced to that entry. For example, next to "Estrogen
Replacement Therapy" it will say "see 'Hormone Replacement Therapy.'" Whenever possible, I have included specific ways to deal with the particular risk factor
and provided toll-free numbers that you can call for further information. The language used in this book is also
meant to be user-friendly. I have found that intelligence
has little to do with a person's understanding of cancer
and the terminology that goes along with it. The people
who are most knowledgeable are those who have had to
be because they themselves or a family member has had
cancer. Therefore, in each entry I have tried to keep the
language simple and approachable. At the back of the
book there is also a short glossary that contains the defi-
nitions of more complex or unfamiliar terms, as well as a
list of books and organizations, many of which provide
toll-free information numbers and free publications.

The list of resource names and numbers I provide fall
into a number of different categories. Many of the organizations listed are solely information organizations that
can supply you with facts that are essential to your health
and well-being. You will also find activist organizations
on the list that are fighting the status quo, pushing for
needed legislation, and raising money for research. These

groups may not help you with your specific illness, but are working on many levels to help empower cancer patients today and make their battle easier in the future. For example, the breast cancer advocacy movement in the early 1990s, which was started by grass-roots groups and became a national movement, made a major impact. It not only focused awareness on this heinous killer of women, but also generated a tremendous increase in funding for research into the cause and prevention of breast cancer. The various advocacy organizations offer you the opportunity to reduce your *risk* of getting cancer in a much broader sense of the word.

You may notice that on several occasions I use the phrase "It could save your life." I use that when I feel particularly strongly about something, such as stopping smoking. I can't say "It will save your life," but there are times when I feel fairly confident that following certain recommendations could do just that. Unfortunately, I can't deliver a wide-brimmed hat to every woman who is going out into the sun or push every woman into a doctor's office for a Pap test or pull cigarettes from mouths. If I could, I would. What I can do is reiterate on these pages what a little commitment and effort can do. I do so when I write that one simple phrase—"It could save your life." So pay attention when you see it, please!

I wish I could say that if you followed every bit of advice in this book, you would not get cancer. I can't. What I can say with some assurance is that the more positive changes you make, the greater chance you'll have of reducing your risk of getting cancer. So whatever you can do to eliminate risk factors in your life could keep you cancer free.

I

Your Body

❧ Abortion

There is some *very limited evidence* that having an abortion may put you at a greater risk of breast cancer. The reasoning behind the theory goes like this. During the first half of pregnancy, increased concentrations of estrogen stimulate breasts to grow, whereas during the second half of pregnancy the breast cells differentiate to allow milk production. If, as some believe, cell termination differentiation (fully matured cells) is protective because it reduces the number of cells in the breast that are susceptible to cancer, when pregnancy is spontaneously aborted or induced, the woman has high levels of estrogen but misses out on cell differentiation, the protective factor. Hence, the increased estrogen puts her at an increased risk. However, the majority of studies show no link between abortion and breast cancer. A review of forty published studies on abortion and breast cancer found no evidence of an increased risk.

❧ *What to do.* The obvious advice on this one is to prevent unwanted pregnancies whenever possible by using contraceptives.

❧ Aerosols

There are many products that come in spray cans: hair sprays, insecticides, furniture polishes, deodorants, cleaners, etc. They are not as dangerous as they once were, since the carcinogen vinyl chloride is no longer used as a propellant. The various fluorocarbons known as Freon, which were known to escape into the upper atmosphere and attack the ozone layer, are also being phased out. The indirect danger to you is the higher risk of skin cancer as the ozone layer, which filters the sun's ultraviolet rays, is depleted. The direct danger is possible inhalation of dangerous chemicals.

🕉 *What to do.*   Do not use aerosols, no matter what propellant is being used. You will be kinder to the earth and may save yourself from problems created by breathing in whatever chemicals are being used.

🕉 *Age*

This is one of those risk factors over which we definitely have no control. On top of that, it is the overall single most important risk factor for cancer! Over half of all cancers occur in people over the age of sixty-five.

🕉 *What to do.*   This information, that the older you get the greater is your risk of cancer, should serve as a little red warning light, reminding you of the importance of following recommended screening guidelines and being aware of body changes that could be a sign of a problem. The earlier any cancer is detected and treated, the better the chance for a cure.

ஜ *Alcohol*

D oes an occasional glass of wine or margarita cause cancer? Probably not. But there have been studies that have shown alcohol's association with some cancers. Even drinking in moderation can be harmful. Moderate drinking for women is defined by the American Cancer Institute, American Institute for Cancer Research, and the Human Nutrition Information Service at the United States Department of Agriculture as one drink a day. (In general, six ounces of wine, twelve ounces of beer, or one ounce of hard liquor is considered a serving.) One study published in 1987 in the *New England Journal of Medicine* found that women who consumed a moderate amount of alcohol increased their risk of breast cancer by approximately 50 percent. What that means is that if your lifetime risk of developing breast cancer was 3.3 percent, your lifetime risk would increase to 5 percent. Another study in the same issue showed an increased risk of breast cancer of 1.5 percent in women who were regular drinkers. A 1992 study at Harvard University and the University of Wisconsin found that women who had two drinks a day had a 50 percent increase in breast cancer risk compared to women who did not drink alcohol. Why can moderate drinking increase a woman's risk of breast cancer? A possible answer is suggested in a small study done at the National Cancer Institute (NCI) by Marsha E. Reichman, Ph.D., in 1993. She found that two drinks a day raised the level of estrogen, a known factor in breast cancer in premenopausal women.

In the late 1950s, a link between alcohol consumption and colorectal cancer was reported by researchers. A report in 1990 contended that just one drink a day raised a person's risk of colorectal cancer by 5 percent.

Alcohol also potentiates the effects of tobacco smoking on cancers of the mouth, pharynx, esophagus, and larynx. Combined exposures to cigarettes and alcohol accounts for 75 percent of all oral and pharyngeal cancers. The risks are greatest with hard liquor or beer rather than wine.

What to do.   If you enjoy some wine or an evening cocktail, you may not want to go on the wagon completely, and that probably isn't called for. But consider cutting down on the amount you consume and the frequency with which you indulge. The key word is *moderation.* (What I find to be a real incentive is thinking of the calories I save every time I don't have a drink.)

Antioxidants

As the name implies, these are substances that act against the harmful effects of oxygen in your body. Antioxidants are found in great abundance in fruits, vegetables, and grains. There has been a lot of speculation and optimism about the positive role that antioxidants may play in the prevention of cancer by neutralizing free radicals. Free radicals, which are formed by the natural process of oxidation, are unstable molecules containing unpaired, highly charged electrons that can damage cells, permitting bacteria, viruses, or other harmful substances to enter the cell. Once there, these electrons can damage the cell's genetic makeup, resulting in cancer. Simply put, free radicals are the bad guys. So having access to antioxidants, which we all do, is of tremendous benefit.

The antioxidant beta-carotene appears to hinder the development of skin cancer and upper digestive-tract cancers, as well as cervical cancer in its earliest stages. Researchers are currently looking into the possible favorable role that vitamins A and E and derivatives of A play in premalignant oral lesions and cancers of the head and neck. Some antioxidants that have their own entries in this book are *beta-carotene, vitamins A, C, E, folic acid,* and the mineral *selenium.*

❧ **What to do.**   Eat foods rich in antioxidants. It can't hurt.

❧ *Artificial Sweeteners*

Get your sweet-tooth craving satisfied without any of the nutritionless calories real sugar supplies. It sounds too good to be true. Is it? No, not necessarily. You needn't rush to the kitchen and toss out those "sugar-free" sodas, cookies, and other items. But you should be aware that there is a possibility that artificial sweeteners might pose a slight risk when it comes to cancer, and keep your consumption of them moderate.

In the late 1960s, amid great public concern (is "panic" too strong?), the Food and Drug Administration (FDA) banned the artificial sweetener cyclamate. Some early studies showed that it caused bladder cancer in laboratory animals, suggesting that we could be similarly affected. Guess what? Results of studies in more recent years have contradicted the initial data on cyclamate. Although it is still banned, the FDA is reviewing the data to see if this artificial sweetener could be considered safe for human consumption and to determine if it should be approved once again for commercial use in restricted amounts.

The elimination of cyclamates did not put an end to artificial sweeteners. The two others currently available are saccharin and aspartame, which is marketed as NutraSweet or Equal. Saccharin was introduced at the turn of the century and has been controversial ever since. In 1907 the chief of the Bureau of Chemistry in the Department of Agriculture expressed concern about it. President Theodore Roosevelt reacted quickly, defending the sweetener. "You tell me that saccharin is injurious to health?" he is quoted as saying. "My doctor gives it to me every day. Anybody who says saccharin is injurious to health is an idiot." Saccharin stayed on the market and continued to grow in popularity.

After some studies linked saccharin with the development of bladder cancer in laboratory animals, the FDA proposed a ban on it again in 1977. That November, Congress passed the Saccharin Study and Labeling Act, which placed an eighteen-month moratorium on any action against saccharin by the FDA. The moratorium has been extended several times. The last extension was to May 1997. The act also required that all foods containing saccharin bear a warning label that read: "Use of this product may be hazardous to your health. This product contains saccharin, which has been determined to cause cancer in laboratory animals." In the late 1970s NCI and the FDA conducted a population study and found, in general, that people who used an artificial sweetener had no greater risk of bladder cancer than people in the population as a whole. However, there was evidence of an increased risk in those people who have six or more servings of sugar substitutes or two or more eight-ounce servings of a diet drink daily. In addition, heavy smokers who used artificial sweeteners had higher rates of bladder cancer than heavy smokers who did not use sugar substitutes. This study is being reviewed by the FDA, and other groups continue to launch their own studies in an effort to more accurately access possible health risks of these substances.

Aspartame, which was introduced in July 1983, has not been shown to cause cancer in laboratory animals.

&ð *What to do.*   Any risk appears to be minimal. As with so many other things, moderation seems the best path to follow if you want to keep using artificial sweeteners. But why not indulge your sweet tooth nutritiously with vitamin-rich, fiber-rich fruits? Substitute fruit juice for some of those diet sodas. And, especially if you use artificial sweeteners, DON'T SMOKE.

&ð *Aspirin*

Aspirin has been shown to reduce the risk of colorectal cancer—IN MEN! Will it help us as well? Who knows. The Physicians Health Study, which began in 1986, tracked 47,900 male health-care professionals. (This is the very same study that looked at aspirin and heart attacks in MEN.) The authors of the study, which was conducted at the Harvard Medical School and Boston's Brigham and Women's Hospital, said that a lower risk for colorectal cancers was found among users of aspirin compared with nonusers. They warned that aspirin should not be recommended as a preventive measure until more is known. Well, I guess we don't have to be concerned with that caution, since we have no way of knowing if aspirin would have the same effect in women as it does with men.

🙤 *What to do.* Check this one out with your doctor. Also, stay on top of what is happening in the medical community regarding the testing of aspirin and its potentially beneficial effects. It is outrageous that an ongoing study of this magnitude does not include women. You might want to let a lawmaker know how you feel about being left out of a medical study whose results could have a major impact on your life.

🙤 *Atypical Hyperplasia of the Breast*

This condition of excessive cell growth, which can show up in a biopsy, moderately increases your risk of breast cancer. It should serve as a warning sign.

🙤 *What to do.* Regular follow-up by your doctor.

ᨒ *Atypical Uterine Hyperplasia*

This condition of excessive cell growth in the lining of the uterus is considered a precancerous condition. Its most common symptoms include heavy menstrual periods and bleeding between periods. Its treatment depends on how severe it is and the age of the woman who experiences it. Young women are usually treated with female hormones and regular observation of the endometrium. In older women who are near menopause or postmenopausal, treatment may be with hormones if the condition is not too severe. In severe cases the usual treatment is removal of the uterus.

ᨒ **What to do.** Regular follow-up by your doctor.

ᨒ *Barbecued Foods*

It's summer and the grill in the backyard is beckoning. What a delight. No stove to make the kitchen even hotter, no pans to scrub. It's quick and easy. And it tastes *sooo* good. Then comes the news that grilling foods could be a risk factor for cancer. Whoops! It turns out that when fatty meats are cooked over a heat source, the fat that drips onto the coals or hot coils form carcinogenic substances. Those substances are then deposited on the food by the rising smoke. The cancer risk posed by barbecued foods appears to be minimal. But it's easy to reduce or eliminate the risk as well.

🌿 *What to do.* Here are some ways to make barbecuing food as healthy as it is good:

BARBECUE HEALTH TIPS

- Meat—When grilling meats, get cuts that are as lean as possible; trim any visible fat before cooking; if frozen, thaw completely to shorten cooking time.
- Fish—Use fish that have a lower fat content, such as haddock, cod, pollack, perch, grouping, whiting, snapper, instead of high-fat fish, such as swordfish, tuna, salmon, anchovy, herring, eel, mackerel, and pompano.
- Make marinades for food from ingredients that contain little or no fat, such as lemon juice, tomato sauce, vinegar, or Worcestershire sauce or rub it with spices.
- Use a rotisserie for more even cooking and to avoid any charring.
- Partially cook food at the stove or in the microwave to reduce the amount of cooking time on the grill and fat that can drip onto the coals.
- Cook over embers and not over flames.
- Put a drip pan on top of the coals to catch fat as it drips from the food being grilled.

Instead of grilling the traditional steak, ribs, or hot dogs—why not switch to vegetables? They are delicious grilled, you don't have to worry about fat, and you get the added bonus of some always welcome vitamins and fiber.

✺ *Beta-carotene*

B eta-carotene is an antioxidant that transforms into vitamin A in the body. It has gotten plenty of hype
over the years and, perhaps, with good reason. One study
done at Johns Hopkins University found that people with
low levels of beta-carotene in their blood were four times
more likely to develop lung cancer than people with
higher levels. In other studies beta-carotene appeared to
offer some protection against breast, uterine, and cervical
cancer. Researchers at the University of Alabama reported that women who ate large mounts of foods containing beta-carotene had lower incidences of cervical
and uterine cancers. Beta-carotene has also been shown
to lower the risk for cancers of the esophagus, stomach,
colon, and mouth.

It appears that beta-carotene can also suppress some
cancers, including uterine and cervical, or even reverse
some cancers, such as precancerous lesions in the mouth.
Beta-carotene is found mainly in fruits and vegetables
that are green or yellow in color.

SOURCES OF BETA-CAROTENE

- apricots
- beet greens
- bok choy
- broccoli
- cantaloupes
- carrots
- egg yolk
- kale
- liver
- mango
- papaya
- peaches
- pumpkin
- romaine, red-leaf, and green loose-leaf lettuces
- spinach

- tomatoes
- turnip greens
- whole milk
- yams
- yellow squash

Studies have indicated, however, that beta-carotene supplements do not have the same effect in the body as equivalent amounts that we get from food we eat. Early in 1996 the National Cancer Institute announced the findings of two major studies that showed that beta-carotene supplements were totally ineffective in preventing cancer or heart disease. NCI head, Dr. Richard Klausner, said that the 40,000 female health professionals who have been taking beta-carotene, vitamin E, and aspirin as part of a third study, would no longer be taking the beta-carotene supplements.

🍠 **What to do.**   Eat a diet rich in beta-carotenes. Stay off those supplements!

🍠 *Birth Control Pills*
see "Oral Contraceptives."

🍠 *BRCA1 Gene*

Although scientists had known of this breast cancer susceptibility gene, it wasn't until 1994 that scientists actually isolated it on chromosome 17 and cloned it. This discovery was heralded as a major breakthrough. It also opened a can of worms. It's estimated that a very small number, only about 5 percent, of all breast cancer cases are caused by this inherited gene. However, if you are one of those who falls into that 5 percent, the news is not good. It appears that more than half the women who have the gene will be diagnosed with breast cancer by the age of fifty and more than 85 percent by age seventy. Having the gene does not guarantee that you will eventually get breast cancer, but it does substantially increase your risk. At present there is no simple test that will show whether you are carrying the BRCA1 gene, although scientists are hard at work to come up with one. An available test will raise more questions, the chief one being: Should you be tested? The information could be more harmful than helpful. If you find out you have the gene, then what do you do? Can you be assured of confidentiality? What happens to your medical insurance if your carrier finds out? Will this be considered a "preexisting condition?" There's no way to get rid of the bad gene or fix it. Your only real options would be regular monitoring by your doctor in order to assure as early detection as possible; or prophylactic mastectomies, which cannot totally eliminate the risk of breast cancer.

ℰ **What to do.**   Nothing yet. But stay on top of this one. It could have many repercussions.

ℰ *Breast-feeding*

If the arguments on how healthy it is for your baby to be breast fed don't sway you, maybe this will. A large study done at the University of Wisconsin in 1994 found that the longer a mother breast feeds her baby and the younger she is when she begins, the more her risk of premenopausal breast cancer decreases. There was no evidence that having breast-fed a baby would reduce the risk of breast cancer in women who are postmenopausal. If that is the case, the number of women who may benefit is relatively small, since menstruating women develop just 20 percent of all breast cancer cases. However, studies in China, where more than half the women breast-feed for at least three years, suggest that long-term breast-feeding reduces breast cancer risk in both pre- and postmenopausal women. Researchers speculate that the reduced risk may be a result of changing hormone secretions, interruption of ovulation, or an actual physical change in the breast.

ஃ **What to do.** If you have no strong feelings one way or the other, go for the breast-feeding. It could benefit you and your baby.

ஃ *Breast Lumps*

When I found a lump in my breast while showering, I nearly died right there of fright. It is without doubt one of the most terrifying things a woman can experience. What I didn't know at the time was that most breast lumps are not cancerous! Of lumps found in the breast, about 80 percent prove to be benign when biopsied. Many women have what is called "generalized breast lumpiness," which is also known as fibrocystic changes, fibrocystic disease, and benign breast disease. The key word here, of course, is *benign.* This condition is not cancer. The biggest problem it presents is that it makes it more difficult to do a breast self-exam. This type of lumpiness usually disappears after menopause.

- Cysts—these are fluid-filled sacs found in the breast and occur most often in women aged thirty-five to fifty. They show up clearly on ultrasound. Your doctor may do a fine-needle aspiration—insert a needle into the cyst and withdraw the fluid—or just watch it.
- Fibroadenoma—this is a tumor that is made up of structural (fibro) and glandular (adenoma) tissue. These are usually sold, round, painless lumps that can be moved around easily. On a mammogram they have a typically benign appearance. Most surgeons think it's a good idea to remove them to make certain they are benign. When I discovered a lump in my breast at the age of thirty-four, it had the characteristics of fibroadenoma—I didn't know the term then—and my gynecologist suggested I do nothing but check it in six months. I insisted on it being removed and it was malignant! This is not typical. But, obviously, it can happen.
- Fat necrosis—these are painless, round, firm lumps formed by damaged and disintegrating fatty tissue. They can result from a bruise or blow to the breast. To be on the safe side, these lumps are surgically removed and a biopsy performed, since fat necrosis can easily be mistaken for cancer.
- Sclerosing adenosis—a condition in which there is excessive growth of tissues in the breast's lobules. A lump caused by this condition frequently causes pain

and occasionally appears as a lump. On a mammogram, it may show up as small deposits of calcium in tissue—calcifications. Adenosis is often difficult to distinguish from cancer, so doctors usually perform a surgical biopsy to diagnose and treat this condition.

• Intraductal papilloma—this is a small wartlike growth that projects into breast ducts near the nipple. A slight bump or bruise can cause it to bleed, resulting in a bloody or sticky discharge from the nipple. The diseased duct can be surgically removed. Multiple intraductal papillomas generally need to be removed.

Will any of these conditions increase your risk of breast cancer? Yes, but on *very rare occasions*. Certain very specific types of microscopic changes in breast tissue do increase risk. These changes feature excessive cell growth, or hyperplasia. Approximately 70 percent of women whose biopsy is benign have no evidence of hyperplasia and are at little or no increased risk of developing breast cancer. About 25 percent of benign breast biopsies do show signs of hyperplasia, including such conditions as intraductal papilloma and sclerosing adenosis. If your biopsies show such hyperplasia, your risk of developing breast cancer is slightly increased. In the other 5 percent of women with benign biopsies, excessive cell growth is found along with abnormal cells. This is diagnosed as atypical hyperplasia and moderately increases the risk of breast cancer.

&❧ **What to do.** Although the risk of benign breast conditions developing into cancer is very small, it certainly warrants further discussion with your doctor on what course to follow.

❧ *Breast Self-exam (BSE)*

This self-screening method is secondary prevention and won't prevent breast cancer, but it could save your life. It probably did for me. I found a malignant lump in my breast when I was thirty-four. I didn't examine my breasts on a regular basis (as I should have) and absentmindedly checked my breasts while showering one day. Although most breast lumps are found by women themselves, there is little data on whether BSE actually reduces mortality. In other words, if you go to the trouble of examining your breasts every month and eventually do find a lump that turns out to be cancer, will you live longer than the woman who never did BSE and whose breast cancer was found by a mammogram or by her doctor? The reason there is no answer is few studies have been done. Cindy Pearson, program director at the National Women's Health Network, says, "Maybe we don't have perfect knowledge about BSE because no one can make lots of money off it, so no one wanted to invest the money to study it." A bit cynical, perhaps, but not without merit.

A study being conducted in Toronto and Finland appears to show that cancer deaths were reduced by BSE. And there is increasing evidence that BSE done correctly can detect a tumor that is relatively small, when there is the greatest chance for a cure. The key word is "correctly." Too often women are not shown how to examine their breasts properly and what to look for. In addition, many women are intimidated or embarrassed by examining their breasts. For a breast self-exam to be effective, you must do it right. Ask your doctor to show you the correct way to perform BSE or go to a women's health center. Breast cancer advocacy groups have sprung up all over the United States. Find one in your area for advice on doing BSE. About a third of the women in the United States practice it monthly, and another half practice it occasionally.

The American Cancer Association recommends that at age twenty women start examining their breasts every month. The best time to examine your breasts is when your period is over and the hormonal stimulation of breast tissue is least apparent. If you are no longer menstruating, choose a day of the month that is significant to you—maybe the date of your birthday—and each month examine your breasts on that day.

<u>DOING A BREAST SELF-EXAM</u>

Step 1. Stand in front of a mirror that is large enough for you to see your breasts clearly. Check each breast for anything unusual. Check the skin for dimpling, puckering, or scaliness. Look for any discharge from the nipples.

Step 2. Watching closely in the mirror, clasp your hands behind your head and check for any change in the shape or contour of your breasts.

Step 3. Press your hands firmly on your hips. Bend slightly toward the mirror as you pull your shoulders and elbows forward and again check for any change in the shape or contour of your breasts.

Step 4. Gently squeeze each nipple and look for a discharge.

Step 5. Raise one arm. Use the pads of the fingertips of your other hand to check the breast and the surrounding area—firmly, carefully, and thoroughly. Some women like to use lotion or powder to help their fingers glide easily over the skin. Feel for any unusual lump or mass under the skin. Feel the tissue by pressing your fingers in small, overlapping areas about the size of a dime. Be sure you cover your whole breast. Take your time and follow a definite pattern: lines, circles, or wedges. It is important to cover the whole breast and to pay special attention to the area between the breast and underarm, including the underarm itself. Check the area above the breast, up to the collarbone, and all the way over to your shoulder.

Step 6. Repeat step 5 while you are lying down. Lie flat on your back, with one arm over your head and a pillow or folded towel under your shoulder. This position flattens the breast and makes it easier to check. Check each breast and the area around it very carefully, using one of the patterns: lines, circles, or wedges.

Step 7. Some women repeat step 5 in the shower. Your fingers will glide easily over the soapy skin, so you can concentrate on feeling for changes underneath.

PATTERNS FOR EXAMINING YOUR BREASTS

Lines: Start in the underarm area and move your fingers downward, little by little, until they are below the breast. Then move your fingers slightly toward the middle and slowly move back up. Go up and down until you cover the whole area.

Circles: Beginning at the outer edge of your breast, move your fingers slowly around the whole breast in a circle. Move around the breast in smaller and smaller circles, gradually working toward the nipple. Don't forget to check the underarm and upper chest.

Wedges: Starting at the outer edge of the breast, move your fingers toward the nipple and back to the edge. Check your whole breast, covering one small wedge-shaped section at a time. Be sure to check the under-arm area and the upper chest.

In her book, *Dr. Susan Love's Breast Book*, the director of the UCLA Breast Center says, "the importance of breast self-exam in the containment of cancer has been greatly exaggerated." She feels the promotion of BSE is misleading and could actually do more harm than good by causing women needless anxiety when they do it—or guilt if they don't do it. She contends that BSE can alien-ate a woman from her body if she is examining her breast as if it were an enemy or hiding a land mine.

Christiane Northrup, M.D., a holistic physician, offers a positive approach to BSE. In her book *Women's Bodies, Women's Wisdom,* Northrup says her advice to her pa-tients is that when doing BSE, "do so *not necessarily to find suspicious lumps* but to send energies of caring and respect to this area of [your] body." Dr. Northrup says if you get to know your breasts and approach them in this way, you'll be surrounding them with a much more posi-tive energy field than the usual one engendered by the BSE, in which you are examining your breasts with dread and fear of what you might find.

🌿 *What to do.*   BSE costs nothing, it is easy to do once you learn how, it takes very little time, and can be done anywhere you have a little privacy. If years from now it is found that it doesn't save lives—well, it cost you nothing. On the other hand, if it does prove to be beneficial, if it saves lives—you'll know you've been doing the right thing. So, do it! For a free publication with instructions on BSE call the Cancer Information Service at (800) 4–CANCER.

᭡ℷ *Broccoli*

T his green-flowered cruciferous vegetable, treated quite disparagingly by former President George Bush, is one of the best cancer-fighting foods we have! It is chock-full of sulforaphane, considered the most powerful anticancer compound known. It is also a good source of calcium, fiber, folic acid, vitamins A and C, and beta-carotene.

᭡ℷ ***What to do.*** Eat that broccoli.

᭡ℷ *Calcium*

R esearchers are evaluating the effectiveness of supplements of the mineral calcium in preventing polyps from recurring in the bowel after they have been removed, because of the strong evidence that colorectal cancer develops from polyps.

SOURCES OF CALCIUM

Milk, cheese, and yogurt (best sources of calcium)
    milk—buttermilk, dry nonfat reconstituted, evaporated, low-fat, skim, whole

cheese—
> best sources: Gruyère, Swiss, Parmesan, Romano, ricotta
> others: blue, brick, Camembert, feta, Gouda, Monterey, mozzarella, Muenster, provolone, or Roquefort

yogurt—plain, flavored or with fruit; made with whole, low-fat, or nonfat milk; frozen

Breads, cereals, and other grain products
> English muffin
> bran muffin
> oatmeal—instant, fortified, prepared
> pancakes—plain or with fruit, buckwheat or whole-wheat
> waffles—bran, cornmeal, wholewheat

Vegetables
> broccoli
> spinach
> turnip greens

Fish
> mackerel—canned, drained
> ocean perch
> salmon—canned, drained

Legumes
> dried beans, peas, and lentils
> tofu

ℬ **What to do.** Although the proof is not yet positive, it can't hurt to make sure you have sufficient amounts of calcium in your diet.

❧ Cellular Phones

I n January 1993 a man from Florida went on a national talk show and claimed that his wife's fatal brain cancer was caused by her constant use of a cellular phone. A short time later, the National Cancer Institute announced that studies were underway to examine the potential risk from the nonionizing electromagnetic radiation released by cellular phones. So far, there have been no "definitive studies" linking cellular phones to brain cancer, and for that reason Dr. Richard Adamson, director of the NCI's division of cancer etiology, says "there is no need to panic."

❧ **What to do.** The studies are continuing, so stay tuned.

❧ Cervical Dysplasia (cervical intraepithelial neoplasia [CIN], squamous intraepithelial lesion [SIL])

T his condition, in which there are abnormal cells in the cervix, can eventually become cancer if not treated. Depending on how much of the cervix is affected and how abnormal the cells are, cervical dysplasia can be low-grade (mild dysplasia or CIN1) with early changes in the size, shape, and number of cells that form the surface of the cervix; medium-grade (moderate dysplasia or

CIN2) with more extensive changes in the cervical cells; or high-grade (severe dysplasia, CIN3) with the greatest number of abnormal cells covering the entire cervix. When it is severe, it may be referred to as cervical cancer in situ, which is the very earliest stage of cancer when it is noninvasive. That means the cancer has not entered or harmed tissue bordering the tumor. It can take many years for the abnormal cells to spread deeper into the cervix and become the far more dangerous invasive cancer.

There are a number of simple ways to remove the abnormal cells without harming nearby healthy tissue. The procedures include cryosurgery, which freezes and kills the cells; cauterization, which destroys the cells through heat; or laser surgery. Removal is considered a cure.

Cervical dysplasia can be found with a Pap test. The American Cancer Society and other organizations recommend that you start getting a Pap test annually when you become sexually active or at age eighteen, whichever comes first. The Pap test is a quick, simple procedure.

ᏅᎦ *What to do.* Since cervical dysplasia can be found by performing a Pap test, it is important to use this screening tool, especially since virtually all cervical cancer that is found early is curable. Get a regular Pap test. It could save your life.

ᏅᎦ *Chemicals*

They're so helpful. They're so hazardous. There are a great number of chemicals that may eventually become estrogenic (act like estrogen) when they enter the body. These can enter your body in various ways: they can come from the foods you eat, the water you drink, and the air you breathe. Chemicals that are estrogenic are found in detergents, cosmetics, condom lubricants, spermicidal foams, pesticides, and other products. But what's the big deal about chemicals acting like estrogen, anyway? Isn't estrogen supposed to be a good hormone? The big deal is that estrogen appears to stimulate some of the gynecologic cancers women get. Some researchers have argued for years that industrial chemicals that adopt estrogenlike effects when in the body contribute to an increased risk of breast cancer. Scientists believe that estrogenic pesticides may affect a woman either through repeated exposure or through exposure during some crucial phase early in her sexual development. Many of the risk factors for breast cancer, for example, are linked to increased amounts of estrogen in the body.

According to Anna Soto, M.D., at Tufts University School of Medicine, the most common hormonal property among chemicals in the environment is their ability to mimic estrogen. She says that there are many of those chemicals out there and they may not be that easy to spot. For example, the chemical nonyl phenol, used in plastics, may contaminate food during processing or packaging. (Soto and her colleague, Dr. Carlos Sonnenschein, M.D., made that serendipitous discovery when they found that plastic they were using in their lab shed estrogenlike chemicals.) Soto and colleagues have developed a test called the E-SCREEN that can measure the estrogenic activity of chemicals. She says that chemicals should be tested for their estrogenic activity before being released into the environment because of the possible hazards of their cumulative effect. And she has proposed a study to see if an increased incidence of breast cancer correlates with the cumulative dose of all estrogenic chemicals in our body.

Studies have found higher levels of chemical pesticide residues in the breast fat of women with breast cancer than in the breast fat of women with benign conditions, according to Ruby Senie, Ph.D., associate attending epidemiologist at Memorial Sloan-Kettering Cancer Center. She says that other studies indicate that exposure to pesticides influences hormonal levels in lab animals.

Research into the biologically active chemicals that accumulate in a woman's body throughout her lifetime is being done by Dr. Mary S. Wolff at the Mt. Sinai School of Medicine in New York. She and her colleagues have compared the breast tissue of women with breast cancer with the breast tissue of women who do not have breast cancer. Wolff says, "These lines of research are fairly unusual, although they seem quite simple and straightforward in terms of the kind of stuff that's out there to be done."

In the mid-1970s consumers in Israel put pressure on the Israeli government to take action against pesticides. The government complied, phasing out the use of organochlorine pesticides at dairy farms. One study found that breast cancer mortality rates dropped overall 8 percent between 1976 and 1986. The authors of the study contend that the true rate of decrease was probably near 20 percent if trends seen before the ban were factored in as well.

❧ *What to do.* This is a tough one. Read product labels carefully. Try to use products that have the least amount of chemicals. Eliminate, to as great an extent as possible, exposure to pesticides. (See "Pesticides in Foods," "Pesticides in Your Home," "Pesticides in the Environment," and "Pesticides on Your Lawn or Garden.")

৯ Chemoprevention

This term refers to the use of natural or synthetic substances to reduce or eliminate the risk of developing cancer. Various chemoprevention studies are being conducted to evaluate the efficacy of different natural or laboratory-made substances to reduce the risk of cancer. Researchers believe that the cancer-prevention agents work by stopping or reversing the process by which a cell becomes malignant. The cell changes that lead to cancer most likely take place in a series of steps over a period of many years, so there may be several points in the process when development can be interrupted.

Participants in a chemoprevention study can be healthy, disease-free people or people at a high-risk of developing a specific cancer or people with cancer who are at risk of developing another cancer. The most widely publicized and controversial study involving women is the Breast Cancer Prevention Trial (BCPT), which is evaluating the hormonal drug tamoxifen for its possible role in preventing breast cancer in women who are at a greater risk than average of developing it. Researchers at the National Cancer Institute have tested or are currently studying various chemoprevention agents. For example, vitamin-A-related compounds have shown promise in preventing cancer of the skin, head, and neck, including the upper airway and food passages, nose, mouth, lips, tongue, gums, cheek, tonsils, pharynx, larynx, esophagus, and lung in people at high risk for these cancers. Researchers are also studying vitamin C. Recent studies indicate that folic acid, a member of the B-complex family, may reduce the growth of precancerous cells in the cervix. And the minerals selenium and calcium are being studied in the prevention of skin and colon cancer, respectively. (See "Tamoxifen," as well as "Beta-carotene," "Retinoids," "Vitamin A," "Vitamin C," "Folic Acid," "Selenium," and "Calcium.")

🏵 *What to do.*   Talk with your doctor about the possibility/advisability of taking part in a chemoprevention clinical trial.

🏵 *Cholesterol-Lowering Drugs*

Since the early 1980s, there has been a tenfold increase in prescriptions for these drugs. In 1992 there were more than 26 million prescriptions for cholesterol-lowering drugs. A study published in the *Journal of the American Medical Association,* in January 1996, found that some of the drugs caused cancer in rodents. Although it is not known if cholesterol-lowering drugs can cause cancer in humans, the findings in the study do raise concern, prompting the researchers to recommend that only people at a high risk of coronary heart disease take the drugs.

🏵 *What to do.*   Of course, talk to your doctor. In addition, why not try to reduce your cholesterol naturally, by cutting the amount of fat in your diet, staying away from foods containing cholesterol, and exercising.

ᵛᵃ *Chronic Obstructive Pulmonary Disease (COPD)*

This is a condition characterized by progressive limitation of the flow of oxygen into and out of the lungs. Emphysema and chronic bronchitis are forms of COPD. People with this condition have a greater risk of developing lung cancer. This condition appears to have a familial association.

ᵛᵃ **What to do.** DON'T SMOKE. Do see your doctor regularly if you have this condition.

ᵛᵃ *Clinical Breast Exam*

This is an examination of your breasts done by your doctor. It is recommended that if you are aged twenty to forty, you get a clinical breast exam every three years; if you're forty years of age or older you should have a yearly clinical breast exam. The National Cancer Institute estimates that over half the women in the United States over fifty do not have a doctor examine their breasts annually. Don't be one of those women! The American Cancer Society recommends that the clinical breast exam be done seven to ten days after your period begins, when your breasts are less lumpy and tender.

🌿 **What to do.**   Having an annual clinical breast exam certainly won't decrease your risk of getting breast cancer. But it certainly might reduce your risk of dying of it if cancer is detected early and treated.

🌿 Clomid
see "Fertility Drugs."

🌿 Coffee

Although too much caffeine may make you jittery and cost you some hours of sleep, it will not cause cancer. Numerous studies have tried to link coffee with a variety of cancers including breast, pancreatic, and bladder but none have been successful.

🌿 **What to do.**   Nothing, really, to reduce your risk of cancer. But if coffee is interrupting your sleep, cut back or go for decaf.

🌿 Cooking Carcinogens

We all know someone who goes to the best steak joint in town and orders the steak "well done, charred." The waiter bristles and admonishes that it is "at your own risk." It turns out there may be a real risk in getting your steak, or any other meat, well-done. When meat is cooked, chemicals can be created that may increase the risk of cancer. For example, carcinogenic chemicals called polynuclear aromatic hydrocarbons (PAH) are formed by burning fat during open-flame cooking. The smoke from the burnt fat contains PAHs that adhere to the surface of the meat. Another class of chemicals known as heterocyclic aromatic amines (HAAs) may also pose a cancer risk. HAAs are created within muscle meats such as beef, pork, fowl, and fish during most kinds of cooking. Based on animal studies, HAAs may increase the number of cancers in the United States in humans by two thousand a year. Now, two thousand cancer cases doesn't sound like a lot, and it isn't, unless you are one of the two thousand. However, it takes very little effort to avoid exposure to HAAs. The most important factor in the development of HAAs is the amount of heat used during cooking. Muscle meats cooked at a temperature over 212° Fahrenheit will produce the greatest percentage of HAAs. Therefore, frying, broiling, and barbecuing produce the largest amounts of HAAs because the meats are cooked at a very high temperature.

What to do. Cook your meats at a lower temperature by oven-roasting, baking, microwaving, stewing, boiling, or poaching to limit your exposure to HAAs.

Copper

A metal . . . that can prevent cancer!? Possibly. Copper is used in your body for healthy tissue development and function. A number of laboratory studies have shown that in a variety of animals certain forms of copper slow the growth of tumors, according to Maria Linder, Ph.D., a professor of biochemistry at California State University in Fullerton. Another researcher, John R. J. Sorenson, Ph.D., a professor of medicinal chemistry at the University of Arkansas, gave copper compounds to mice, then administered fatal doses of radiation. Half survived. He says the copper protected the mice from the harmful effects of the radiation.

Copper is easy to include in your diet. It's present in a lot of foods, including navy beans, avocados, liver, crabmeat, nuts and seeds, wholewheat foods, apricots, bananas, and chicken. One precaution, too much vitamin C in your diet could interfere with copper absorption.

🥣 *What to do.*   In a varied diet, eat some foods that contain copper.

| 🥣 *Crohn's Disease*

This disease usually appears during young adulthood and seems to run in families. It produces chronic inflammation that may involve any part of the digestive track. Those who have it may experience problems with absorbing nutrients, which could result in deficiencies in calcium, vitamin B_{12}, and folic acid. People with Crohn's disease are at a higher risk of developing colorectal cancer.

🥣 *What to do.*   You should be examined regularly by a doctor.

ᛒᚨ *Cruciferous Vegetables*

A friend of mine, looking over my shoulder as I was working on this book, asked rather sarcastically, "What is cruciferous?" I answered (pleasantly) that cruciferous refers to plants with cross-shaped flowers and pointed pods and are named for their likeness to a crucifer—one who bears a cross. Cruciferous vegetables contain sulforaphane, which is considered a powerful anticancer compound. Researchers at Johns Hopkins University found that sulforaphane blocks tumor growth in rats treated with a cancer-causing agent. In other studies of rats, regular meals of the actual vegetables had the same effect. Sulforaphane is considered one of the most powerful anticancer compounds found in food. Its major source is broccoli.

Cruciferous vegetables are also rich in the anticancer chemical indole-3-carbinol. In animals it can reverse breast cancer. In humans indole-3-carbinol produces changes in estrogen metabolism that are consistent with protection from breast cancer. Indoles also appear to be effective in protecting against other forms of cancer, including that of the stomach and the large intestine.

CRUCIFEROUS VEGETABLES

beet greens	kale
bok choy	kohlrabi
broccoli	mustard greens
brussels sprouts	radish
cabbage	rutabagas
cauliflower	turnip greens
collard greens	turnips

Research has also shown other promising anticancer compounds in cruciferous vegetables. Some seem to stimulate the release of enzymes that act against cancer. Most cruciferous vegetables are good sources of fiber. Some, mainly kale, collard greens, and turnip greens, are a good source of calcium. Brussels sprouts provide iron.

🍃 **What to do.**   Eat that broccoli . . . and other cruciferous vegetables.

🍃 Cyclamate
see "Artificial Sweeteners."

🍃 DDT (dichloro-diphenyl-trichloroethane)

The pesticide DDT, discovered in 1939 and introduced in the United States in 1945, was viewed as a miracle until its great potential for harm was seen. It was banned in the United States in 1972 because it had become ubiquitous in the food chain, has a long half-life, and posed a threat to humans as well as the insects it was meant to destroy. More than two decades after DDT was banned, residues remain in the environment (and in the bodies of many women).

DDT is one of a number of pesticides that can mimic estrogen and produce estrogenic effects in the body. If the theory is true that as estrogen in the body increases so does a woman's risk of breast cancer, then exposure to pesticides (which end up as estrogen in fatty breast tissue) may very well be a significant risk factor in the development of breast cancer.

In a 1992 pilot study Dr. Frank Falck Jr., at the University of Michigan, found that the breast tissue in women with breast cancer had 50 to 60 percent greater concentrations of contaminants such as PCB and pesticides such as DDT (an organochlorine) than the breast fat tissue of women without breast cancer.

Breast surgeon Alison Estabrook compared levels of DDT in the blood and cysts of women with gross cystic disease at Columbia Presbyterian Hospital in New York. Estabrook found higher levels of DDT in the fluid of breast cysts than in the blood, as well as higher levels of estradiol (a potent form of estrogen) and other substances. Estabrook notes that Long Island, New York, which has elevated levels of breast cancer, was a farming community that used DDT to spray crops, and that even if it hasn't been used in twenty years, the residue might still affect the drinking water.

When food contaminated with the pesticide DDT is eaten, the residue accumulates in the fatty tissue of the breast and stays there forever. If DDT is a factor in the development of some breast cancers, the women at the greatest risk are those women who had the greatest exposure to DDT when it was being used in the United States from 1945 until it was banned in 1972. Hence, DDT may be one of the factors accountable for the sharp rise in breast cancer in women over fifty on Long Island, since they would fit right into that category.

Another pesticide under investigation is endosulfan. Endosulfan enters the food supply as a pesticide on carrots, lettuce, spinach, tomatoes, and other crops. A study by the Environmental Working Group, a private organization, found that two million pounds of endosulfan are applied to crops each year. According to researcher Anna Soto, endosulfan has as potent an estrogenlike effect as DDT. Soto found that estrogenic pesticides accelerated the reproduction of breast cancer cells and that different estrogenic pesticides, such as endosulfan, dicofol, and methoxychlor, accumulate together as if they were the same chemical. If that's true, estrogenic pesticides that are not banned are potentially adding to the banned pesticides such as DDT that are still in a woman's body.

Studies looking at environmental factors like DDT have not been well supported for a variety of reasons. One is the male medical establishment's skepticism that they pose a risk; another is the companies that produce various suspect products denigrate the idea of possible problems. A study published in 1993, comparing the levels of DDE (a by-product of DDT) in the blood of women with breast cancer and women without breast cancer, found women with the highest levels of DDE in their blood were four times as likely to have breast cancer as those women with the lowest levels.

Another study, published in 1994, did not support the hypothesis that DDT is associated with breast cancer. The author of that study acknowledged that more research is needed to clarify the relationship, if there is one, between DDT and breast cancer. Research is continuing. The organization Silent Spring Institute, in Boston, is studying residents on Cape Cod. Of the ten towns in Massachusetts with the highest breast cancer rate, seven are on Cape Cod. In New York the National Cancer Institute is conducting a study on Long Island, because of the elevated breast cancer rates there. Researchers are tracking women's exposure to DDT as well as other environmental pollutants.

ஃ **What to do.**   Although there is nothing you can do to undo exposure to DDT, endosulfan, or other pesticides, there are precautions you can take to prevent or limit exposure in the future. (See "Pesticides in Foods," "Pesticides in Your Home," "Pesticides in the Environment," and "Pesticides on Your Lawn or Garden" for easy precautionary steps to take.)

ஃ *Decaffeinated Coffee*   *Tea?*

I n 1976 trichlorethylene (TCE), a chemical being used to remove the caffeine from coffee, was found to cause liver tumors in mice. After the National Cancer Institute published that information, companies that had been using TCE switched to methylene chloride (dichloromethane) or other chemicals to decaffeinate the coffee.

ஃ **What to do.**   If you drink decaf and want more information on the chemicals being used in decaffeination, call the Food and Drug Administration at (202) 205–4317. You may also want to call or write the company that makes the brand you use to inquire about what method of decaffeination they use.

ዮ *DES (diethylstilbestrol)*

D ES is a synthetic hormone that acts like estrogen. It was one of the first synthetic estrogenlike hormones that was inexpensive and could be taken orally. It was developed in 1938 and prescribed for women from 1945 to 1971 to prevent miscarriage. In 1971 a link between DES and cancer of the female reproductive system was discovered and the Food and Drug Administration issued a warning that DES should not be used during pregnancy. A small number of adolescent girls whose mothers had taken DES-type drugs during pregnancy developed a very rare cancer of the vagina called clear cell adenocarcinoma. Daughters whose mothers took DES may have a higher risk of developing cervical cancer as well.

ዮ *What to do.*   While there is no way you can change the fact that your mother took DES, by being aware of the possible risk at which it puts you, you can take extra precautions by making sure you have an annual Pap test. You should also talk with your doctor about it.

ዮ *Diet*

A lthough today there are articles galore on foods to eat and not to eat to avoid cancer, diet's role in cancer has been a topic of research for a relatively short period of time. In 1974 diet and cancer research at NCI started with a budget of less than 3 million dollars. In

1990 the budget had grown to more than 67 million dollars.

Dr. Peter Greenwald, director of the National Cancer Society's division of cancer prevention and control, says that by eating a diet rich in fruits and vegetables you could cut your risk of getting cancer to half that of people who eat smaller amounts. He is not alone in that opinion. In its landmark report *Diet, Nutrition, and Cancer,* published in 1982, the National Academy of Sciences states that diet is responsible for 60 percent of women's cancers. Reducing fat intake to no more than 20 percent of total calories and increasing fiber to 25 to 30 grams a day could prevent more than 150,000 cancer deaths a year. That thinking is echoed by a number of authorities on cancer nutrition.

BASIC DIET GUIDELINES

- Eat a variety of foods, such as fruits and vegetables; whole-grain breads and cereals; lean meats, poultry and fish; dried peas and beans; and low-fat dairy products. You cannot get all the nutrients you need from one food.
- Maintain your ideal weight. Obesity, which is defined as 40 percent above your ideal weight, has been linked with some cancers.
- Avoid too much fat, saturated fat, and cholesterol. A diet low in fat may reduce the risk of breast, colon, and rectal cancer.
- Eat foods with adequate starch and fiber, such as fruits, vegetables, potatoes, whole-grain breads and cereals, and dried peas and beans. A diet high in fiber reduces the risk of colon and rectal cancer.

- Avoid too much sugar. Sugar has lots of calories and is of virtually no nutritional value.
- Avoid too much salt, which may contribute to high blood pressure.
- If you drink alcohol, do so in moderation. Alcohol has been associated with cancers of the mouth, throat, esophagus, liver, and breast. Drinks with alcohol are also high in calories and low in nutritional value.

U.S. Agriculture Department's Daily Food Guide

FOOD GROUP	SUGGESTED ½ CUP SERVINGS
Vegetables	3 to 5
Fruits	2 to 4
Breads, cereals, rice, pasta	6 to 11
Milk, yogurt, cheese	2 to 3
Meats, poultry, fish, dried beans and peas, eggs, nuts	2 to 3

🍃 *What to do.* Following those recommendations not only will reduce your risk of cancer but will reduce your risk of many other diseases as well. (The following risk-reduction factors related to what you eat have their own entries: antioxidants, barbecued foods, beta-carotene, coffee, cooking carcinogens, cruciferous vegetables, fat, fiber, fish oil, folic acid, food preparation, fruit, garlic, green tea, herbs, iron, milk, olive oil, retinoids, selenium, soy, vegetables, and vitamins A, C, and E.)

❧ *Digital Rectal Exam*

I n this exam, your doctor inserts a lubricated, gloved finger in the rectum to check for any abnormality on its wall. This is a screening test for colorectal cancer that the American Cancer Society recommends be done on a yearly basis once you turn forty. As many as 15 percent of all colorectal cancers arise in tissues that can be felt by a doctor performing a digital rectal exam.

❧ *What to do.* Although some people feel uncomfortable getting this test, and you may be one of them, it is quick, painless, and could save your life by detecting colorectal cancer early, when it is most curable.

❧ *Dioxin*

D ioxin is a toxic chemical that is produced by incinerators, chemical processing, chlorine bleaching of paper and pulp, and the burning of diesel fuel. In 1994 the EPA said that to date, dioxin could be responsible for anywhere from 26,500 to 265,000 cases of cancer and that even minute amounts of dioxin might trigger a variety of health problems, including uterine cancer. A panel of scientists criticized the conclusions of the study because of the "scientific methodology" that was used. Dioxin was also used in the defoliant Agent Orange in the Vietnam War.

❧ *What to do.* One of the greatest sources of dioxin is meat. Here is one more reason to reduce the meat in your diet.

✆ *Diuretics*

Diuretics are prescribed for conditions such as hypertension (high blood pressure), certain heat conditions, and edema (excess fluid in the body's tissues) to increase urine flow. They may also increase your risk of developing kidney cancer. A study in the middle 1990s found women who had taken diuretics faced nearly three times the risk of renal cell, or kidney, cancer compared to women who did not take the drug. The author of the study, Joseph McLaughlin, at the National Cancer Institute, acknowledged that the results were, "too preliminary to advise any changes for patients taking prescription diuretics," adding that not all studies have shown this connection. This is one to definitely not panic over—and to definitely discuss with your doctor if she wants to prescribe it for you.

✆ *What to do.* Look at other nonmedical ways of reducing fluid in your body, such as reducing or eliminating salt from your diet.

✆ *Dry Cleaning*

In 1995, a survey in New York City of a dozen apartment buildings which housed dry cleaning establishments found the air in most of the apartments to contain levels of the dry cleaning solvent perchloroethylene (perc) exceeding the recommended limit for long-term exposure. In eight of the apartments the level was ten times the standard set by the state. The actual risk to long-term tenants is not known. If you don't live above a dry cleaner you may still face a risk. According to a report by Consumers Union in 1996, even wearing dry-cleaned clothes can be hazardous. The study published in *Consumer Reports* measured consumer exposure to perc and found levels in freshly dry-cleaned clothing high enough for concern. Dr. Edward Groth III, an environmental scientist who took part in both studies, said that over the long term, "consumers who wear a lot of dry-cleaned clothes can be exposed to a significant increase in cancer risk" from the carcinogen perc.

 What to do.   I've avoided as much as possible buying clothing that require dry cleaning because of the expense of dry cleaning and the inconvenience. You may want to reduce any possible risk and, at the same time, save some money by following suit. When you do get clothes dry-cleaned, remove the bag and hang the clothes in an out-of-the-way place so they can air and any perc residues can dissipate. Consider going to a dry cleaner who uses a water-based process instead of perc. And only dry-clean clothes that must be dry-cleaned and that actually need to be cleaned.

Endometrial Hyperplasia

This is a condition in which an overabundance of cells are lining the uterus. It is generally considered a precancerous condition. Although it does not always result in endometrial cancer, it always precedes its development. Symptoms of endometrial hyperplasia may include heavy bleeding during menstruation, erratic bleeding between periods, or abnormal or heavy bleeding during menopause.

🙽 **What to do.**   If you are experiencing those symptoms, see your doctor. An endometrial aspiration or D & C can be used to diagnose the condition. If it is hyperplasia, removal of the tissue in those diagnostic procedures will remove the risk of cancer.

🙽 Endosulfan
see "DDT."

🙽 Erythroplakia
(erythroplasia)

This condition in the mucous membrane of the mouth, in which a reddened patch appears, is considered a precancerous condition for oral cancer. The most common site in women is the gums. It is associated with heavy smoking and drinking and develops most often in people aged sixty to seventy. Erythroplakia is the most common and earliest sign of oral cancer.

🙽 **What to do.**   See your doctor or dentist, and limit your alcohol consumption, and DON'T SMOKE.

✳ *Estrogen*

E strogen, the name for a group of steroid hormones that control female sexual development, has long been implicated in the development of breast cancer. In the late eighteenth century, the English physician Sir George Thomas Beatson was the first to control the spread of breast cancer by removing the woman's ovaries, her primary source of estrogen.

In the female body estrogen is produced primarily by the ovaries. A small amount is secreted by the adrenal glands. Estrogen can be bad or good. It breaks down into either a stronger, long-lasting form that is bad, or a weaker, short-acting type that is good. Although there is substantial evidence that estrogen can increase the risk of breast cancer, the exact role it plays has not been defined and is still being investigated. There are a number of different theories.

Richard Theriault, M.D., at M.D. Anderson Cancer Center in Houston, says that there is no data to suggest that estrogen is an initiator of breast cancer or that it is itself a carcinogen. He does say, however, that it is likely that estrogen promotes the cancer once it has developed.

In the 1970s Harvard epidemiologist Brian MacMahon did a study in which he concluded that the following factors, all of which result in a prolonged, uninterrupted presence of high estrogen levels in the body, put a woman at an increased risk:

- The younger a woman is when she starts menstruating (in the last two hundred years, the age of menarche has declined dramatically; in 1860 it was seventeen and in the early 1990s it was twelve).

- The older a woman is when she has her first child.
- The older a woman is at menopause (women who start menopause at fifty-five or older have twice the risk of breast cancer as those with menopause before forty-five).

Two other risk factors are believed to be the length of time between menarche and first pregnancy, the longer the time, the greater the risk, and not having any children.

&❧ **What to do.** There is nothing you can do to avoid these risk factors other than having children, and at an earlier age, which is obviously not a practical solution. However, if you do have those risk factors, you may want to discuss it with your doctor and come up with a plan for greater surveillance.

❧ Estrogen Replacement Therapy
see "Hormone Replacement Therapy."

❧ Exercise

Exercise has been prescribed for losing weight, reducing stress, lowering your risk of heart disease, and just plain staying fit. Now it appears that exercise may reduce your risk of some cancers. That is good news, because exercise, like diet, is something over which we have control. The bad news is that most of us, some 60 percent, lead sedentary lives, according to the Centers for Disease Control and Prevention (CDC).

There are several ways that exercise may reduce our risk of developing cancer. Research has shown that moderate exercise will result in an increased amount of natural killer (NK) cells in your body, which are then more active as well. Natural killer cells are a type of white cell that contains potent chemicals. They attack tumor cells and infected body cells. Normal cells are not affected by them. Natural killer cells are thought to play a major role in cancer prevention by destroying abnormal cells before they have a chance to pose a real threat. A study in 1990 found that exercise more than tripled the level of natural killer cells in the blood of the participants.

Exercise promotes contraction of the bowel. When contraction is increased, waste products are excreted more rapidly, reducing opportunities for carcinogens and the colorectal lining to make contact. This reduces the risk of colorectal cancer.

Finally, exercise may reduce your risk of ovarian, uterine, and breast cancer by lowering the levels of hormones in the body that can stimulate abnormal cell growth leading to cancer. High levels of exercise in young women can delay the start of menstruation, cause longer cycles, or halt ovulation altogether, thereby lessening exposure to crucial hormones. A study reported by Harvard researchers in 1981 found that college-age women athletes were less likely to develop breast cancer than those who did not exercise regularly or strenuously.

Leslie Bernstein, Ph.D., at the University of Southern California, found that regular exercise during the reproductive years can substantially lower breast cancer risk. In studies Bernstein discovered a continued protective effect from such exercise as regular ballet dancing, running, or swimming, which delayed the onset of menses, and noticed a continued protective effect from exercise among women aged twenty-five to forty.

Another advantage exercise offers is weight control. Obese women are at a greater risk of ovarian, breast, and uterine cancer because fatty tissue releases estrogen. Obesity may be a risk factor in other cancers as well, including colorectal and kidney cancer.

The obvious questions are, how much exercise, and what kind, is enough? Unfortunately there is not an obvious answer. In 1985 the American College of Sports Medicine (ACSM) recommended twenty minutes of aerobic exercise—activity intense enough to produce a sweat—three times a week. In early 1995, ACSM and the Centers for Disease Control issued new, more time-consuming and less strenuous recommendations, advising adults to perform a total of thirty minutes of moderate-intensity exercise—no sweat—daily. These recommendations were a result of analyzing major studies and coming up with a program that would be beneficial and at the same time feasible. Several months later, an analysis from the Harvard Alumni Health Study (all MEN!!) indicated that moderate exercise was not enough—you had to sweat. Although fewer exercise studies have been conducted on women than on men (read this line several times until your blood is boiling), most have indicated that moderate exercise has decided benefits.

🎵 *What to do.*   Why, exercise, of course—unless for medical reasons you cannot. Besides the possibility of reducing your risk of some cancers, you'll get all those other advantages already mentioned. While you can join a fancy gym, that is certainly not necessary. Exercise can be done at home or at a local park at no cost whatsoever. There are some very simple things you can do on a daily basis to get a little more exercise: take the stairs instead of the elevator, park at the farthest end of the parking lot at the mall, get off the bus or subway a stop or two earlier. Another possible bonus—once you get into it, it may go from being a chore to fun.

🎵 Familial Adenomatous Polyposis (FAP)

This is a rare, inherited condition, affecting about one person in eight thousand. It is a disease in which multiple polyps, often several hundred, develop throughout the colon during adolescence and early adulthood. Between one half to two thirds of untreated people with familial polyposis develop colorectal cancer during their forties and fifties. By the time they reach fifty-five, the probability of their having colorectal cancer is nearly 100 percent.

🎵 *What to do.*   If you have this condition, you should be regularly monitored by a doctor.

℘ Familial Atypical Multiple Mole Melanoma (FAMMM) Syndrome

This is a family tendency to develop the skin cancer melanoma. It was first recognized as a hereditary cancer in 1820, when an English surgeon diagnosed this disease in several members of the same family.

℘ **What to do.**   If you have this syndrome, you should be checked regularly by your dermatologist or regular doctor.

℘ Family History

see "Heredity."

℘ Fat

There is more and more evidence that eating too much fat may increase your risk of getting various cancers, including breast, uterine, ovarian, skin, pancreatic, and colon. For example, the United States, Great Britain, and the Netherlands, countries in which the consumption of fat is high, have among the highest breast cancer rates, whereas in Japan, Singapore, and Rumania, where a very lean diet is eaten, the incidence of breast cancer is one sixth to one half the rate in the United States. Dr. Larry Norton, M.D., head of the breast and gynecological medical service at Memorial Sloan-Kettering Cancer Center in New York, says that the epidemiological evidence is clear-cut, that countries with high-fat diets and high calorie diets have more breast cancer.

In 1991 researchers at the University of Toronto said that a study involving some 56,000 women found that the risk of developing breast cancer rose in relation to the amount of fat in the diet; that every 77 grams, or 693 calories, of fat consumed a day increased a woman's risk of breast cancer 35 percent. The study also found evidence that a woman whose fat intake represented 47 percent of her daily calories was 50 percent more likely to develop cancer than one who limited her fat intake to 31 percent of calories a day.

A study done at Yale University and published in 1994 found that for every ten grams of saturated or animal fat a day that a woman consumes, her risk of ovarian cancer rose 20 percent. Fat consumption has also been associated with prostate and colon cancer. In Greece researchers found that people with colon cancer had eaten fattier foods than people without colon cancer, and that those who ate the most meat and the least vegetables had eight times the risk of getting colon cancer. A Canadian study found that a high-fat diet more than doubled a person's risk of getting it.

Best Sources of Low-Fat Food

FOOD	SERVING	CALORIES	FAT GRAMS
DAIRY PRODUCTS			
Cheese:			
low-fat cottage (2%)	½ cup	100	2
mozzarella, part skim	1 oz	80	5
parmesan	1 tbs	25	2
Milk			
low-fat (2%)	1 cup	125	5
nonfat, skim	1 cup	85	trace
Ice Milk	1 cup	185	6
yogurt, low-fat, fruit flavored	1 cup	230	2
MEATS			
Beef			
lean cuts, such as trimmed bottom round, braised or pot-roasted	3 oz	190	8
lean ground beef, broiled	3 oz	230	16
lean cuts, such as eye of round, roasted	3 oz	155	6
lean and trimmed sirloin steak, broiled	3 oz	185	8
Lamb			
loin chops, lean and trimmed, broiled	3 oz	185	8
leg, lean and trimmed, roasted	3 oz	160	7
Pork			
cured, cooked ham, lean and trimmed, roasted	3 oz	135	5
center loin chop, lean and trimmed, broiled	3 oz	195	9
rib, lean and trimmed, roasted	3 oz	210	12
shoulder, lean and trimmed, braised	3 oz	210	10

FOOD	SERVING	CALORIES	FAT GRAMS
Veal			
cutlet, braised or broiled	3 oz	185	9

POULTRY

FOOD	SERVING	CALORIES	FAT GRAMS
Chicken, roasted			
dark meat without skin	3 oz	175	8
light meat without skin	3 oz	145	4
Turkey, roasted			
dark meat without skin	3 oz	160	6
light meat without skin	3 oz	135	3
Egg			
hard-cooked	1 lge	80	6

SEAFOOD

FOOD	SERVING	CALORIES	FAT GRAMS
flounder, baked, no butter or margarine	3 oz	85	1
oysters, raw	3 oz	55	2
shrimp, boiled or steamed	3 oz	100	1
tuna, packed in water, drained	3 oz	135	1

OTHER FOODS

FOOD	SERVING	CALORIES	FAT GRAMS
salad dressing, low-calorie	1 tbs	20	1

LOW-FAT SNACK SUGGESTIONS

Fresh and dried fruit	Fresh vegetables	Breadsticks
Finn Crisp	Flatbread	Graham crackers
Hardtack	Matzo	Oyster crackers
Pretzels	Popcorn (air-popped)	Rusks
Ry-Krisp	Saltines	Soda crackers
Swedish crispbread	Wasa Brod	Zwieback toast

Source: U.S. Department of Agriculture.

So how much fat should you eat? David Rose, M.D., chief of the division of nutrition and endocrinology at the American Health Foundation, says, "We believe the percentage for risk is a maximum 20 percent of fat. . . . We have to reduce fat to that level to get benefit."

❧ **What to do.** If your diet is higher than 20 percent fat, lower your fat consumption.

| ❧ Fecal Occult Blood Test
see "Occult Blood Stool Test."

| ❧ Fertility Drugs

Taking certain fertility drugs may increase your risk of developing ovarian cancer, especially if you do not become pregnant. A study published in 1994 gave further credence to earlier studies that had suggested a connection between the use of fertility drugs and the development of ovarian cancer. According to the study, the drug clomiphene, which is sold under the brand names Clomid and Serophene, increased risk 2.5 times if used for longer than a year. Dr. Alice Shittemore, of Stanford University, calls that increased risk "substantial." The researchers found that the ovarian tumors that developed were generally of low malignant potential. They respond better to treatment than the more common type of ovarian cancer. No increased risk was found in women who had been on the fertility drug human chorionic gonadotropin (HCG).

The *PDR Guide to Women's Health and Prescription Drugs* describes the ovarian hyperstimulation syndrome (OHSS) in which the ovary is enlarged. It has occurred in women on clomiphene and may progress rapidly and become serious.

EARLY WARNING SIGNS AND SYMPTOMS OF OHSS

- severe pelvic pain
- nausea and vomiting
- weight gain
- abdominal pain
- abdominal enlargement
- diarrhea
- difficult or labored breathing
- less urine production

If you are taking Clomid or Serophene and are experiencing any of the above symptoms, see your doctor immediately.

Studies into fertility drugs and ovarian cancer are continuing.

– *What to do.* For more information on fertility drugs call (301) 496–5133 or write to the Office of Research Reporting, National Institute of Child Health and Human Development, Building 31, Room 2A32, Bethesda, MD 20892. You can also contact the individual drug companies that manufacture the drug. Marion Merrell Dow Pharmaceuticals of Kansas City, MO, sells Clomid; Serono Laboratories of Norwell, MA, sells Serophene.

✿ *Fiber*

Fiber, which is also referred to as roughage or bulk, is the part of vegetables, fruits, and grains that are not digested by the body when eaten. Numerous studies have shown that increasing fiber intake (and decreasing fat consumption) substantially lowers the risk of developing colorectal cancer. It's not known just why fiber is so beneficial, but there are some theories. Increased fiber in the diet results in greater stool bulk and more rapid movement of the stool through the colon, so the concentrations of any carcinogens in the stool and the amount of time they are in contact with the bowel may be reduced. In addition, increased fiber may change the chemical composition of the stool. The National Cancer Institute estimates that if every American ate 20 to 30 grams of fiber each day, there could be a 50 percent reduction of colon cancer.

Fiber may also be a factor in breast cancer. In Finland the fat intake is similar to that of women in the United States, the rate of breast cancer is not. Finland has a lower rate of breast cancer; however, their fiber consumption is much higher than the fiber intake of women in the United States. That suggests that fiber may play a role in reducing the risk of breast cancer as well. Fiber appears to reduce levels of circulating estrogen, which may promote the growth of breast tumors.

BEST SOURCES OF FIBER

- Foods with 6 or more grams of fiber per 1 ounce serving: Extra Fiber Bran cereal (14), All-Bran (9–10), 100% Bran (9–10), and bran, unsweetened.

NEXT BEST SOURCES OF FIBER

- Breads and cereals with 4 grams per 1 ounce serving: Bran Chex, Corn bran, Cracklin' Bran, raisin bran, and wheat germ (toasted or plain).
- Legumes, cooked, with 4 grams per ½ cup: kidney beans, lima beans, navy beans, pinto beans, and white beans.
- Fruits with 4 grams: ½ cup blackberries, and 3 dried prunes.

Sources with 1 to 3 Grams of Fiber Per Serving

FOOD	SERVING
BREADS AND CEREALS	
bran muffins	1 med
popcorn (air-popped)	1 cup
whole-wheat bread	1 slice
whole-wheat spaghetti	1 cup
40% Bran Flakes	1 oz
Grape-Nuts	1 oz
granola-type cereals	1 oz
Cheerios-type cereals	1 oz
Most	1 oz
shredded wheat	1 oz
Total	1 oz
Wheat Chex	1 oz
Wheaties	1 oz
LEGUMES (COOKED) AND NUTS	
chickpeas (garbanzos)	½ cup
lentils	½ cup
*almonds	10
*peanuts	10

FOOD	SERVING

VEGETABLES

artichoke	1 small
asparagus	1/2 cup
bean sprouts	1/2 cup
beans, green	1/2 cup
broccoli	1/2 cup
brussels sprouts	1/2 cup
cabbage, red and white	1/2 cup
carrots	1/2 cup
cauliflower	1/2 cup
celery	1/2 cup
corn	1/2 cup
green peas	1/2 cup
kale	1/2 cup
parsnip	1/2 cup
potato	1 med
rutabagas	1/2 cup
spinach	1/2 cup
summer squash	1/2 cup
sweet potato	1/2 med
tomato	1 med
turnip	1/2 cup

FRUITS

apple	1 med
apricot, dried	5 halves
apricot, fresh	2 med
banana	1 med
blueberries	1/2 cup
cantaloupe	1/4 melon
cherries	10
dates, dried	3
figs, dried	1 med

FOOD	SERVING
grapefruit	1/2
orange	1 med
peach	1 med
pear	1/2 cup
pineapple	1/2 cup
raisins	1/4 cup
strawberries	1 cup

*high in fat, use with discretion
Source: National Institutes of Health

ᢞ **What to do.** You should be eating at least 25 grams of fiber a day. If you are eating less, build up to the 25 grams gradually to avoid harmless but unpleasant side effects such as flatulence and bloating.

| ᢞ *Fish Oil*
see "Omega-3 Fatty Acid."

| ᢞ *Flaxseed*

Flaxseed may have been among the first crops planted for food some ten thousand years ago by Romans and Egyptians. It's a regular part of the diet of some African countries. It has been touted for its ability to lower cholesterol. And now it appears it may play a role in the prevention of cancer. Flaxseeds are an important source of lignans which have been known, since the 1940s, to be antimitotic (inhibit cell division and growth). Drugs used to treat cancer are mainly antimitotics. Some animal studies have suggested that the lignans in flax-seeds may interfere with the development of breast, prostate, colorectal, and other cancer tumors. Today, flaxseed is often added to multigrain breads and cereals, muffins, cookies, and breakfast bars.

🪶 ***What to do.***   Although the data on the possible benefits of flaxseed is very preliminary, adding it to your diet can't hurt. You can find flaxseed flour or meal in some stores. Another source is flax oil, which has a nutty flavor and is good in stir-fry cooking. Whole flaxseeds will keep for several months in cool, dry storage. For more information on flaxseeds and even some recipes, call the Flax Council of Canada at (800) 817–9894.

🪶 *Folic Acid (folacin)*

This member of the B-complex family, which occurs in food as folate, may reduce your risk of colorectal cancer, cervical dysplasia, and carcinoma in situ in the cervix. People with a deficiency of folic acid have higher rates of stomach and esophageal cancer. Folate is required for DNA metabolism and plays a role in such genetic functions as cell division and tissue growth. Chromosome damage is believed to be a significant part of the process that causes malignancy. One theory holds that folate can repair chromosome damage, thereby preventing the development of cancer; or it may prevent a cancer-causing gene from switching on.

The best sources of folic acid are braised beef or calf liver, chicken, turkey, black-eyed peas, and cooked lentils. Other sources include: artichoke, asparagus, beets, broccoli, brussels sprouts, cauliflower, Chinese cabbage, corn, endive, chicory, escarole, romaine, mustard greens, okra, parsnips, dried beans and peas, lima beans, kale, spinach, turnip greens, grapefruit and orange juice, whole-wheat English muffin, whole-wheat pita bread, ready-to-eat fortified cereals, plain wheat germ, and crabmeat. (See also "Chemoprevention.")

෯ *What to do.* Include foods in your diet that provide folic acid.

෯ *Food Preparation*

The way you prepare food for cooking and cook it can reduce possible hazards.

FOOD PREPARATION AND COOKING TIPS

- Trim all visible fat from meats before and after cooking.
- Remove skin before cooking chicken.
- Broil, poach, or roast meats, and drain the fat from the pan.
- Substitute broth for grease in cooking main dishes and accompaniments.
- Use spray shortenings and butter substitutes.
- Use nonstick cookware to avoid extra fat.
- Season meats, fish, and vegetables with herbs, spices, or lemon juice.

෯ *What to do.* With very little effort you can make the food you eat healthier. If you are not already following the above suggestions—phase them in.

❧ *Fruit*

I n your diet of at least five fruits and vegetables a day,
you should have more vegetables than fruits. The following chart is a simple way to see quickly which fruits
provide the greatest source of vitamin A, vitamin C, vitamin E, fiber and folate:

Benefits

FRUIT	AMT	A	C	E	FIBER	FOLATE
apple	1 med		*	*	*	
apricot	1/2 cup	*		*	*	
apple juice	3/4 cup		**			
apricot nectar	1/2 cup	*				
banana	1 med	*			*	
blackberries	1/2 cup		*		*	
blueberries	1/2 cup		*		*	
cantaloupe	1/2 cup	*	**			
cranberry juice	1 cup		**			
dates	1/4 cup				*	
grapefruit	1/2 med		**			
grapefruit juice	3/4 cup		**			
grapefruit/orange juice	3/4 cup		**			
grape juice	3/4 cup		**			
guave	1				*	
honeydew	3/4 cup		**			
kiwi	1 med		**		*	
mandarin orange sections	1/2 cup	*	**			
mango	1/2 med	**	**		*	
nectarine	1 med	*	*	*	*	
orange	1 med		**		*	
orange juice	3/4 cup		**			

FRUIT	AMT	A	C	E	FIBER	FOLATE
papaya	¼ med		**			
peach	1 med		**			
peaches, dried cooked	½ cup				*	
peaches, dried uncooked	¼ cup				*	
pear	1 med		*		*	
pineapple	½ cup		**			
pineapple juice	¾ cup		**			
plum	1 med		*			
pomegranate	1 med		*			
prunes, dried cooked	½ cup				*	
prunes, dried uncooked	¼ cup				*	
raisins	¼ cup				*	
raspberries	½ cup		*		*	
strawberries	½ cup		**		*	
tangelo	1 med		**		*	
tangerine	1 med		**			
watermelon	1¾ cup	*	**			

🌿 **What to do.** Besides providing lots of vitamins and other essential nutrients and fiber, fruits make great snacks and are a good choice when you just feel like having something sweet.

🌿 *Gardner's Syndrome*

This is a very rare inherited condition in which multiple polyps are found in the colon. It occurs in about one in 14,000 births and carries with it a greatly increased risk of colorectal cancer and possibly pancreatic cancer. Between one half to two thirds of untreated people with Gardner's syndrome develop colorectal cancer during their forties and fifties. By the time they reach fifty-five, the probability of their having colorectal cancer is nearly 100 percent.

🍂 **What to do.** If you have this condition, you should see a doctor regularly.

🍂 Garlic

There may be good reasons besides taste for ordering extra garlic on that pizza. Ancient Egyptians fed garlic to their slaves to keep them healthy. Romans gave it to their soldiers and workers. It is believed that Hippocrates (c. 460–c. 377 B.C.) used garlic to treat uterine cancer.

Researchers are investigating garlic for its possible role in preventing and fighting cancer. It appears that garlic is toxic to some cancer cells. In a study done by the National Cancer Institute in China, the people who had eaten the most garlic and onions (53 pounds a year) were 60 percent less likely to have stomach cancer than those who had rarely consumed those foods. Garlic and onions contain chemicals called allylic sulfides, which appear to activate enzymes that neutralize cancer-causing substances. Scientists are beginning to isolate and identify some one hundred compounds found in garlic.

🍂 **What to do.** For the latest information on garlic, call the Garlic Information Center at the New York Hospital-Cornell Medical Center in New York. It has set up a garlic hot line at (800) 330–5922.

℘ *Green Tea*

W ouldn't it be loverly if you could prevent cancer by drinking a cup or two (or three or four) of tea (specifically green) a day? The main ingredient in green tea that appears to give it its cancer-fighting reputation is an antioxidant called epigallocatechin gallate or EGCG. In 1994 the National Cancer Institute released findings of studies on people and animals in Shanghai. It concluded that green tea could reduce the incidence of cancer of the esophagus. Studies in Japan have shown lowered rates of lung, stomach, and skin cancers. But, alas, most of the data, impressive as it is, is from animal studies. Animals given green tea (or EGCG in water) have developed fewer tumors of the skin, lung, esophagus, stomach, small intestine, colon, liver, pancreas, and breast. Chung S. Yang, an expert on tea and cancer at Rutgers University in New Jersey, says, "Tea is impressive because it inhibits such a wide spectrum of cancers." You would not have to drink gallons of tea to reap benefits either. Yang says that the green tea cuts tumor rates when given to animals at levels that approximate what humans would drink. In addition, it appears to inhibit tumors at different stages of growth—when they're just beginning or when they're proliferating. Most researchers, though, say it's too early to encourage people to stock up on green tea.

Green tea is the least processed tea, the youngest and freshest. In Asian countries it is held in high esteem. It is thought to purify the body, delight the senses, and lift the spirits. Green tea is delicate in color and flavor. When brewing it, hot but not boiling water is poured over the leaves. The brewing time is just a minute or two. Boiling water is too harsh for green tea, as is the addition of milk or sugar.

🍃 **What to do.**   Green tea is not harmful and may do some good. But be sure not to have it steaming hot. Repeated scalding of your throat could cause damage to your esophagus, which could result in cancer.

🍃 *Hair Dyes*

I f you dye your hair, *a lot,* you may want to give it a little more thought. A study by the American Cancer Society and the U.S. Food and Drug Administration, published in 1994, found that women who use permanent hair dyes do not have an overall increased risk of dying from cancer, although women who used black hair dyes for more than twenty years had a slightly increased risk of dying from non-Hodgkin's lymphoma and multiple myeloma. Over the years, various studies have shown an association between hair dyes and an increased risk for ovarian cancer, multiple myeloma, non-Hodgkin's lymphoma, and leukemia. It is thought that the hair dyes may contain chemicals that can alter the structure of DNA and cause cancer in animals. The amount of these chemicals, and their structure, vary from product to product. Darker dyes tend to have greater amounts of the chemicals than lighter dyes. Some of the substances in hair dyes are easily absorbed through the skin and scalp during application. Most of the risk appears to be associated with permanent and semipermanent dyes used over a long period of time. A 1993 study at the Harvard School of Public Health and the University of Athens Medical School found that women who used hair dyes five or more times per year had twice the risk of developing ovarian cancer as did women who never used hair dyes. Because the evidence from the studies of personal use of hair dyes is not conclusive, no recommendation to change hair dye has been made by the International Agency for Research on Cancer, the organization that classifies exposures as carcinogenic to humans.

&a *What to do.* If you do use permanent hair dye, be aware of the possible hazards.

&a *Hereditary Nonpolyposis Colorectal Cancer (HNPCC) (Lynch syndromes I and II)*

This is a rare inherited condition. People with Lynch syndrome I are at a very high risk of developing colorectal cancer at a young age—under fifty. People with Lynch syndrome II are at an increased risk of developing a number of different cancers besides colorectal, including uterine, ovarian, small bowel, stomach, and pancreatic at an earlier age than these cancers usually occur.

&a *What to do.* If you have this syndrome, your condition should be followed regularly by your doctor.

᪣ Heredity

The significance of a family history of cancer was not really documented until the late nineteenth century when a worried woman told a doctor she expected to die of cancer. Her reason for coming to this dire conclusion was that virtually all her relatives had died of cancer. The doctor, Alfred Scott Warthin, began to study two generations of her family. In 1913 he published his groundbreaking paper, "Heredity with Reference to Carcinoma as Shown by the Study of the Cases Examined in the Pathological Laboratory of the University of Michigan, 1895–1913." Warthin concluded, "A marked susceptibility to carcinoma exists in the case of certain family generations and family groups." Unfortunately, the woman who inadvertently prompted his historic study did die of cancer as she had predicted she would.

Today we are quick to worry if many family members have had cancer. But should we? Having a relative or relatives who had a specific cancer does not mean you will automatically get it. The family factor may give you a predisposition, which may or may not be realized. Whether it does depends, to some extent, on your behavior and environmental factors. Knowing that you may be at an increased risk of developing cancer should make you more vigilant about limiting your exposure to anything that might increase that risk, and about making your lifestyle as healthy as possible.

Heredity plays a role in a number of different cancers, including ovarian cancer, breast cancer, melanoma, colorectal cancers, leukemia, and possibly lung and brain cancer.

If you have immediate family members—a mother, sister, daughter—who have had ovarian cancer, you are at a greater risk of developing it. The risk is especially high if two or more close relatives have had the disease. The risk is not quite as high for women who have only more distant relatives—grandmother, aunt, cousin—who have had ovarian cancer. However, studies have shown that most women with risk factors do not develop the disease and many women who do get ovarian cancer have none of the risk factors.

Although the role of heredity in colorectal cancer is not fully understood, it appears that 5 to 7 percent of colorectal cancers may be affected by heredity. Among family members of patients with colon cancer, the risk of developing it is three to four times greater than it is in the general population. Women in some families with colorectal cancer have an added risk of developing cancer of the uterus! The risk is greatest when two or more first-degree (immediate) relatives have it. In families where it occurs at an unusually young age, children are at a much greater risk of developing the disease.

Researchers have discovered several genes in the development of polyps and cancer that appear to be defective versions of genes that normally control cell growth. It is believed that these genes can be inherited and present at birth or can develop after birth, spontaneously or under the influence of carcinogens. There are several known genetic conditions involving colon polyps that are known to increase the risk of developing the cancer. Familial polyposis is one. It is a rare, inherited disease in which multiple polyps, often several hundred, develop throughout the colon during adolescence and early childhood. Between one half and two thirds of people with familial polyposis, if untreated, will develop cancer by the time they are fifty-five. It affects one person in 8,000. Gardner's syndrome is similar to familial polyposis. It involves multiple polyps of the colon along with other non-cancerous growths, usually in the skin, jaw bones, and skull. It affects one person in 14,000. Two other syndromes are Turcot's syndrome and Oldfield's syndrome.

Melanoma can run in families. Having two or more close relatives who have melanoma increases your risk. Ten percent of all patients with melanoma have family members who also have had it.

Breast cancer can also run in families. The mothers, daughters, and sisters of women with breast cancer, especially if the relative developed this cancer at a young age (before menopause), are two to five times more likely to develop breast cancer. A family history of prostate cancer may also be a risk factor for breast cancer. David E. Anderson, Ph.D., at M.D. Anderson Cancer Center in Houston, says that "studies indicate a genetic association between prostate cancer and breast cancer that is independent of other hereditary cancers." And it apparently works the other way around.

Your increased risk may be less than you think. When 150 women, at a higher risk of breast cancer than the average woman, were asked what they thought their risk was, they believed it was five to ten times higher than the 6 percent that it actually was. All women have a one-in-eight chance of developing breast cancer during their lifetime. Women with a first-degree relative with breast cancer have a one-in-seven or one-in-six risk. The degree of risk depends on a number of factors, including the type of cancer and the number of affected relatives.

The inheritance of a strong ability to metabolize the

chemical debrisoquine (found in cigarette smoke) is thought to be a risk factor for the development of lung cancer.

If you think you are at a greater risk for a particular cancer because of your family history, you may want to go for genetics counseling to find out if you really are at an increased risk and if so, how great that risk is.

✌ *What to do.*

STEPS TO TAKE IF YOU HAVE A FAMILY
HISTORY OF CANCER

- Know the warning signs for that cancer.
- Discuss with your doctor screening methods and how often they should be done.
- Avoid, to as great an extent as possible, any factors that could increase your risk.
- Consider prophylactic surgery: this is an extreme solution and generally used only in cases of the highest risk. If you are thinking about this, be sure to get a second opinion.
- Let other family members know if you have a hereditary cancer, so that they can take preventive measures.

To find a genetics counselor near you, ask your doctor or call the National Cancer Institute's Cancer Information Service at (800) 4–CANCER. You cannot change your family history. But you can use it to help detect cancer as early as possible. Believe it or not, this cloud does have a silver lining. Knowing that you have an increased risk gives you the opportunity for increased vigilance, which could be life saving.

✍ *Homosexuality*

L ifestyle factors appear to put gay women at greater risk of developing breast cancer, according to epidemiologist Suzanne G. Haynes at NCI. She collected surveys that had been done on lesbians that asked about factors known to put women at a greater risk of developing breast cancer. Haynes concluded that lesbians have a two to three times greater risk of breast cancer than heterosexual women.

A statement from the NCI, following the release of Haynes's statement in 1993, said that Haynes's conclusions were based on an analysis of factors known to increase the risk of breast cancer, including not having children or having them after the age of thirty, and heavy drinking. Dr. Ed Sondik, deputy director of the NCI's Department of Cancer Prevention and Control (DCPC), says, "There is no evidence that being a lesbian intrinsically increases the risk." There is actually very little evidence of any kind on breast cancer in the lesbian population because at that time no study had been done measuring the actual incidence and mortality from breast cancer in lesbians.

Katherine A. O'Hanlan, M.D., associate director of the Gynecologic Cancer Service at Stanford University School of Medicine, agrees that demographic information about the population is "entirely lacking." But that is just one part of a much more global problem, much of which involves the rights and treatment of gay women. O'Hanlan says studies document homophobic attitudes among many doctors and nurses. These homophobic attitudes are often perceived by patients and, as a consequence, a lesbian may stop going for yearly exams or for screenings out of concern that she will not receive the best treatment or simply out of discomfort. In one survey, 94 percent of the lesbians who responded agreed with the statement, "You'd get poorer care if they knew you were [gay]." Forty percent agreed with the statement, "It's like putting your life in someone's hands who really hates you." Any woman, regardless of sexual orientation, who does not go for breast screening regularly (clinical exams and mammography) is at a greater risk of having breast cancer diagnosed when it is more advanced and therefore less likely to be treated successfully.

There is evidence that many lesbians internalize the oppression they experience, according to O'Hanlan. As a result they are more likely to overeat (be overweight), smoke cigarettes, and drink more than heterosexual women. These are all risk factors for breast cancer. Factors such as overeating, drinking in excess, smoking, and limited doctor visits, which may be linked to the oppression lesbians experience, are risk factors that can be turned around.

A position paper on health care was passed by the American Medical Women's Association in 1993. Among other things it called for recognition by all health-care providers that homophobia is a health hazard and that "sensitivity to lifestyle and sexuality issues should be present in the interview, examination, diagnosis, and treatment of lesbian, gay, and bisexual patients."

What to do. If you are gay and have risk factors such as overeating, drinking in excess, or smoking, eliminate them to as great an extent as possible. If you feel your doctor is homophobic, find a doctor with whom you are comfortable.

⌘ *Hormone Replacement Therapy (HRT)*

Curse or cure? Sorry, there's no easy answer on this one. HRT has been shown to increase the risk of breast and endometrial cancer. It also lowers the risk of heart disease and osteoporosis and relieves some common side effects of menopause, such as hot flashes. In June of 1995 the latest study results from the ongoing Harvard University Nurses' Health Study showed that women who take hormones at menopause for five or more years face an increased risk of developing breast cancer. After reviewing some twenty-four studies and three meta-analyses, in 1992 Dr. Janet Henrich of Yale reached the conclusion that "in women who use estrogen for short periods of time, most of the evidence indicates that there is not an increased risk of breast cancer." She and several other experts say women can take estrogen for five years and perhaps longer without putting themselves at higher risk for breast cancer.

It appears that the length of time a woman is on HRT may be the key. Various studies have shown a 25 to 50 percent increase in risk of breast cancer in women who are on it for fifteen or twenty-five years. It appears that, overall, per year of HRT there's a 3 percent increase in breast cancer risk, whereas normally there is a 2 percent increase per year in women during the postmenopausal period. The women at greatest risk are those with a family history of breast cancer.

Another unanswered question is whether women who have had breast cancer can ever take estrogen. Since estrogen appears to be a factor in the development of breast cancer, estrogen is generally not prescribed for women who have had the disease, out of concern that the estrogen will lead to a recurrence. However, it's not known which would be most beneficial to women with breast cancer: withholding estrogen therapy and putting them at a greater risk of heart disease and osteoporosis, or giving them estrogen therapy and increasing their risk of breast cancer and decreasing the risk of heart disease and osteoporosis. A woman who is a long-term survivor of breast cancer has competing risks of mortality: breast cancer recurrence, heart disease, and osteoporosis. Although it has been customary not to prescribe HRT for any woman who has had breast cancer, a group of doctors have questioned the assumption that it would put a woman at risk of recurrence, saying there was little data either way.

There are an increasing number of women who are going into early menopause because of cancer treatment, and there is also concern about the menopausal side effects that result, as well as the increased risk of osteoporosis and heart disease for those women.

Heavy use of HRT is a factor in the development of endometrial cancer if the estrogen is not combined with progesterone or a similar compound called progestin. Initial findings in the Postmenopausal Estrogen/Progestin Interventions (PEPI) Trial, to test the effects of HRT, were published in the *Journal of the American Medical Association* in 1995. The study found that one third of the women taking only estrogen developed endometrial hyperplasia, a potentially precancerous condition. The addition of progesterone appears to eliminate any increased risk of endometrial cancer.

℘ **What to do.** To make a decision, you must weigh the possible increased risk of breast cancer against the well-documented health benefits of estrogen therapy, including lowering the risk of heart disease (which kills far more women than breast cancer) and osteoporosis and increasing blood levels of HDL, the "good" cholesterol. Many researchers contend that the benefits of hormone replacement therapy outweigh the risks for most women.

WAYS TO LIMIT POTENTIAL HAZARDS WHILE TAKING HRT

- Do a breast self-exam every month.
- Get a yearly mammogram.
- Get a yearly physical exam.
- Get a yearly Pap test.

℘ Human Papillomaviruses (HPVs)

There are over seventy types of HPVs, which cause warts. In most cases the warts are annoying but not harmful. They can grow on hands, feet, the mouth, and in the genital area. Genital HPVs can be transmitted sexually—through intercourse, oral or anal sex. Although most genital warts do not cause cancer, there are some that could cause cervical cancer. Some types of HPVs are more carcinogenic than others and are classified as low-risk, moderate-risk, and high-risk. A small percentage of women with certain types of abnormal cells caused by HPVs will develop cancer if the cells are not removed.

Women at the greatest risk of getting an HPV and developing cervical cancer are those who started engaging in sexual intercourse at an early age or have multiple sexual partners.

And here's just one more reason to stop smoking. Cigarette smoking increases the risk that cancer will develop.

&a **What to do.** HPV is one risk factor that is fairly easily controlled with frequent Pap tests and careful medical follow-up. And DON'T SMOKE.

&a *Hypertension*

This is a risk factor for endometrial cancer.

&a **What to do.** Get treatment, and discuss with your doctor ways to monitor for early detection.

&a *Infertility Drugs*
see "Fertility Drugs."

&a *Inflammatory Bowel Disease (ulcerative colitis)*

This disease can cause rectal bleeding, diarrhea, dehydration, fever, anemia, and an elevated white blood cell count. If you have had this condition for ten years or more involving most of the large intestine, your risk of colorectal cancer increases.

🕭 **What to do.**   If you have inflammatory bowel disease, you should see a doctor regularly to have your condition monitored.

🕭 Lynch Syndrome

see "Hereditary Nonpolyposis Colorectal Cancer."

🕭 Mammography

To mammogram or not to mammogram . . . that is the question. Although one would assume the answer would be a simple "yes," it's not that easy.

Mammography, taking an X-ray picture of the breast, is currently the best way of screening for breast cancer. It has been touted for years. So why is there so much controversy about it? Because, like so many things, mammography can have both good and bad consequences.

"The Good News": Mammography can detect small lumps before you or your doctor can feel them, leading to earlier detection of this deadly disease. (The earlier breast cancer is detected and treated, the better the chance for a cure.) A mammogram can also show areas of calcifications or other changes in the breast that can be an indication of possible problems. Mammograms save lives. Studies have well established that mammography

saves the lives of many women over the age of fifty and that thousands of more lives could be saved if all women age fifty and over got regular mammograms. Dr. Larry Norton, head of the breast and gynecologic medical service at Memorial Sloan-Kettering Cancer Center, says, "If everybody did what they're supposed to with mammograms, probably the breast cancer death rate would drop by about 30 percent." Mammography is safe. Progress in technology has improved their accuracy and reduced the level of radiation you are exposed to during a mammography, thereby virtually eliminating any possible risk of cancer as a result of the radiation. There is now a federal law requiring quality FDA standards for mammography facilities.

"The Bad News": A false negative can give a woman a false sense of security, whereas a false positive will likely lead to a lot of anxiety and an unnecessary biopsy. There are many of both. Studies have failed to conclusively demonstrate that mammography lowers the mortality rate in women under the age of fifty, as it does in older women. At the time when the Clinton administration was working on a health plan, breast surgeon Susan Love, director of the UCLA Breast Center, commented that if she were setting up the plan, "I wouldn't pay for mammograms [for women] under fifty for screening." Mammograms can be expensive, and many women find them so painful that they will not get another. Mammograms are described as possibly giving some discomfort.

In the mid-1990s the National Cancer Institute got up on the fence and said it was no longer in the guidelines business and would not recommend who should get a mammogram and when. At the same time, the American Cancer Society and others stuck with their recommendation that women between the ages of forty and forty-nine get a mammogram every other year and that women fifty and older get an annual mammogram. Some doctors say that it is more important for women under the age of fifty to get a mammogram every year, because breast cancer that develops before menopause appears to be more aggressive than postmenopausal breast cancer.

🍃 *What to do.* It's not easy to know which way to go when even the experts disagree. The best thing to do is talk to your doctor about mammography and keep an eye out for breaking news stories regarding this screening method. For information on where you can find an FDA certified mammography facility call the NCI's Cancer Information Service at (800) 4–CANCER.

🍃 *Menopause*

E arly menopause or oophorectomy (removal of the ovaries) at an early age, which results in a virtual absence of estrogen, has a marked protective effect for breast cancer. A woman who stops ovulating at age thirty-five has about a 70 percent reduction in her lifetime risk of breast cancer. Larry Norton, M.D., at Memorial Sloan-Kettering Cancer Center in New York, says that women who are born without ovaries and don't produce estrogen have essentially no breast cancer, or such a low incidence of breast cancer that it's in the range of less than 1 percent of the incidence of normal women with intact ovaries. And he says that when breast cancer cells are studied in the laboratory, their stimulation by estrogen can be seen.

🐟 *What to do.* This is one of those risk factors over which we have no real control. If you go into menopause at a late age, mid-fifties or older, be aware that this is considered a risk factor for breast cancer, and be sure to get a yearly mammogram, do monthly BSE, and get a yearly clinical breast exam. These are things all post-menopausal women should be doing anyway!

🐟 Milk

When researchers at Roswell Park Memorial Institute in Buffalo, New York, compared the risk of drinking whole milk to the risk of drinking fat-reduced milk (2 percent or skim), they found fewer cases of cancer among patients who drank fat-reduced milk.

But there's another possible problem with milk. Early in February 1994, the drug bovine somatotropin (BST), a milk-production stimulant, went on sale. It is the first economically important product of genetic engineering to be used in farming in the United States. It can raise a cow's output of milk 5 to 20 percent. It has also raised considerable controversy.

John Shumway, a dairy producer in upstate New York, told the Wisconsin Farmers Union that he stopped using BST after thirty-four of his two hundred cows developed mastitis, a potentially severe udder infection. A dairy farmer in Michigan reported that two of his cows had died after he used BST.

Monsanto, the drug's manufacturer, said that in the first six months of sales it received ninety-five complaints about BST from dairy farmers, including of the deaths of thirty-six cows. John O'Hara, an FDA spokesman, said that the rate of deaths reported in BST-treated cows was lower than would be expected among the cow population in general.

However, Dr. Samuel Epstein, professor of occupational and environmental health at the School of Public Health at the University of Illinois, says BST could potentially put a woman at greater risk of breast cancer. He claims there is evidence linking milk from treated cows with an increased risk of breast cancer. He charges that the FDA has ignored that evidence. The hormone induces an increase in an insulinlike growth factor, IGF-1, in cow's milk. Epstein says that IGF-1 promotes the transformation of normal breast epithelium to breast cancer. Epstein says he has notified both the FDA and NCI of his concerns.

According to the FDA, "The suggestion that IGF-1 in milk can induce or promote breast cancer in humans is scientifically unfounded and misguided." The FDA says that the milk from treated cows has not been found to be different from the milk of untreated cows.

&ε **What to do.** Since you get the same nutrients in fat-free milk—calcium, riboflavin, and vitamins A and C—as you do in whole milk, it makes a lot of sense to go with skim milk. It just takes getting used to.

If you're concerned about IGF-1 being in your milk, ask your grocer whether the milk being sold in that grocery is from cows who were on the hormone. If the grocer does not know, demand that he find out. The FDA does not require that information to be included on the carton. So, it may take some effort on your part to find out. However, it is also important to note that there is no definitive proof that IGF-1 in your milk will increase your risk of cancer.

ஓ *Moles*

I t is normal to have between ten and forty moles, areas of the skin that contain a cluster of melanocytes. You can develop new moles from time to time, but generally you'll only get new ones until the age of forty. Congenital moles, the ones you are born with, carry a greater risk of becoming malignant than the new ones. But most moles do not become cancerous and will begin to disappear as you age.

A typical mole has symmetrical borders and a uniform color that can range from pink to dark brown or black. About one in ten people have at least one unusual, or atypical, mole that looks different from an ordinary mole. Moles that are not ordinary are called dysplastic nevi. They are more likely to turn into a melanoma than an ordinary mole. However, having a dysplastic mole does not mean you will get melanoma. What it does mean is that it should be checked by a doctor.

SUSPICIOUS MOLE CHANGES

- change in the shape of the mole from symmetrical to asymmetrical—one half is shaped differently from the other
- an irregular border with edges that are ragged, blurred, or notched
- an uneven color, or color that changes over time

- a diameter of over a quarter of an inch
- hardening or softening, a change in the mole's consistency
- scaling, crusting, or bleeding—any obvious change in the surface of the mole
- pain, soreness, or itching
- skin surrounding the mole that becomes reddened or sore looking

🔊 **What to do.** If you do have moles, check your skin regularly and see a doctor immediately if you see any suspicious changes in a mole.

🔊 Mouthwash

A study by the National Cancer Institute found a possible connection between mouthwashes with a minimum of 25 percent alcohol and oral and pharyngeal cancer. NCI and the FDA feel the data are too preliminary to issue a warning. Dr. Clifford Whall, director of product evaluations for the American Dental Association, agrees that further studies are needed.

🔊 **What to do.** I don't need further studies to make sure my mouthwash is under 25 percent alcohol.

✒ *Nitrates, Nitrites, and Nitrosamines*

N itrates and nitrites are chemicals that are added to some cured meats and cheeses as a preservative. Nitrates spontaneously turn into nitrites at room temperature and then they combine with normal bacteria in the mouth. When nitrites combine with other compounds containing nitrogens (are you still with me?), nitrosamines can be formed—and they're the bad guys. At one point, the FDA considered banning the use of nitrates and nitrites in foods. Now the FDA regulates their use and has lowered the amounts that may be used in food. In addition, vitamin C and other nitrosamine-inhibiting substances are now routinely added to salt-cured and smoked foods. Nitrates and nitrites are commonly found in salt-cured foods like bologna, ham, hot dogs, and sausage; smoked foods, including chicken, turkey, salmon, and tuna; and salt-pickled foods, such as tongue and pickles. Exposure to nitrates, nitrites, and eventually nitrosamines increases your risk of developing stomach and esophageal cancer.

✒ *What to do.*   Nitrates and nitrites are listed on food labels—so check labels. You don't have to go "cold smoked-turkey," but if you are a big bacon, hot dog, and sausage eater, you may want to cut back on your consumption of those foods. The key word here is *moderation.*

❦ *Obesity*

I f you are over your ideal weight by 40 percent, you are considered obese and you are 160 percent more likely to die of cancer than another woman who is not. Because fatty tissue releases estrogen, your risk of breast, ovarian, and uterine cancer rises, since estrogen can stimulate abnormal cell growth in these organs, eventually resulting in cancer. So if you know you are overweight, it's not just for appearance's sake that you should be losing weight. Women who are 50 pounds overweight are nine times as likely to develop endometrial cancer as women of normal weight. When excess fatty tissue turns certain hormones into a form of estrogen, you are at a greater risk of endometrial cancer. You are twice as likely to develop this cancer as women who are of normal weight.

Women who have been obese before going into menopause are at a decreased risk of developing breast cancer. The reason may be that young obese women tend to ovulate less frequently and therefore have lower estrogen levels and less exposure to the hormone. However, that advantage is short-lived. In addition, the number of premenopausal women who get breast cancer is significantly lower than postmenopausal women. Postmenopausal women who are obese are at an increased risk of breast cancer. Their risk rises because body fat itself produces estrogen. So when hormonal levels are decreasing in women because of ovulatory cycle decline during and after menopause, excess body fat may become more important. Walter Willett, M.D., professor of medicine at Harvard Medical School, says these innate biological processes may account for the different risk levels, and not fat intake per se.

Obesity may also be a risk factor in ovarian, colorectal, and kidney cancer.

🙠 *What to do.* Take off that extra poundage. No, it's not easy. But it is something over which you have control. Some exercise will help.

🙠 *Occult Blood Stool Test (fecal occult blood test; stool guaiac test)*

This is a safe, simple, inexpensive screening test for colorectal cancer. The test is to find hidden (occult) blood in a stool sample, which could be an indication of cancer (as well as many other conditions, such as hemorrhoids, ulcers, polyps, or other noncancerous conditions). In a number of screening programs, fewer than 10 percent of positive test results were caused by cancer. On the other hand, false negative results can occur because some tumors bleed intermittently or too little to be detected. Studies are being done to determine if mass screening of the general public with the occult blood stool test can reduce the death rate from colorectal cancer. In the meantime, it is recommended that the test be done yearly once you turn fifty.

🙠 *What to do.* Do it. It can't hurt. And if colorectal cancer is found early, treatment could save your life.

✺ Olive Oil

O live oil is rich in unsaturated fatty acids. In Greece, where the incidence of breast cancer is lower than in the United States, 2,300 women took part in a study conducted by the University of Athens and the Harvard School of Public Health. The researchers found that women who consumed olive oil at more than one meal a day had a significantly lower risk of breast cancer than the women who used olive oil less frequently. The study results were published in the January 18, 1995, issue of the *Journal of the National Cancer Institute*.

 ✺ *What to do.*   When you are going to use an oil in cooking or in a salad dressing, use olive oil.

✺ Omega-3 Fatty Acid

T his is a fish oil rich in polyunsaturated fat. It is looked upon by many as a "wonder" oil. The healing powers attributed to it by many include the ability to protect against heart attacks, high blood pressure, and the inflammatory responses in the body that cause such illnesses as arthritis and psoriasis. It may also reduce the risk of various cancers, including breast, ovarian, uterine, and colorectal.

Omega-3s appear to inhibit the hormone estrogen or breast cancer cells. Studies of mammary tumors in animals found that diets containing 20 percent fish oil resulted in reduced tumor incidence and delayed onset of chemically induced tumors.

Sources of Omega-3

FISH (3½ OUNCES, COOKED)	OMEGA-3 GRAMS
anchovy, European canned	2.1
herring, Atlantic	2.1
salmon	1.3
pollack	1.5
grouper	1.3
mackerel	1.3
swordfish	1.1
oyster	1.0
whiting	0.9
trout	0.9
mussel	0.8
eel	0.7
halibut	0.6
crab, blue	0.5
rockfish	0.5
perch	0.3
shrimp	0.3
clam	0.3
haddock	0.2
cod	0.2

🐟 **What to do.**   You should have a minimum of two to three servings a week of foods containing omega-3. What *not* to do: take fish-oil supplements. When the possible benefits of fish oil were extolled, suddenly fish-oil supplements surfaced and multiplied. There are several reasons to be wary.

• There are still many unanswered questions about the effectiveness, safety, and best amount of fish oil. Potential long-term side effects have not been sufficiently researched.

- Fish oil's anticlotting effect can be dangerous if you are in an accident or undergoing surgery; it can also increase the risk of a stroke.
- Fish oil in liquid or in capsule form, such as cod liver oil, may contain pesticides or other contaminants.
- Cod liver oil is overly rich in vitamins A and D, which can be toxic in doses that are too high.
- Too much fish oil could result in a vitamin E deficiency.
- There is no evidence that fish-oil supplements provide the same benefits as eating fish.

℘ Oral Contraceptives

Oral contraceptives, better known as the "pill," first became available to women in the United States in the 1960s. They have been the source of health-related questions and controversy ever since. As of 1994, some 11 million women in the United States were taking the pill. There is no question that the pill is effective as a contraceptive. There is a major question as to whether it can cause cancer. It has been linked with several.

In the mid-1980s several studies reported an increased risk of breast cancer among young women, under the age of forty-five, who had used the pill at a relatively young age, generally before age twenty-five or before their first pregnancy. Around the same time, a report from the Centers for Disease Control and Prevention (CDC) said its investigation showed no increased risk of breast cancer overall or in any specific subgroup. However, a reanalysis of the data in the CDC study did show a subgroup, childless women, who were at an increased risk of breast cancer. Concern over the possibility that the pill might put some women at an increased risk of breast cancer prompted more research. A study in Boston, reported in the *American Journal of Epidemiology* in February 1989, showed higher risk with increasing number of years of use of the pill. However, it also found an increased risk for short-term users and did not find the risk limited to women who started to use the pill at a very young age. A study published in April 1994, at the Fred Hutchinson Cancer Research Center in Seattle, found an increased risk for breast cancer among women under the age of thirty-five who took the pill for more than ten years, and the study supported other evidence that long-term use of oral contraceptives may increase the risk for the early onset of breast cancer. The researchers found that women under thirty-five who used oral contraceptives for more than ten years had a 70 percent increased risk of breast cancer compared to women who had never taken them or had taken them for less than one year. In addition, they found that women who took the pill within five years after they started menstruating faced a 30 percent increased risk. A study headed by researchers at the National Cancer Institute, published in June 1995, added more evidence that early use of the pill increased the risk of breast cancer in women under the age of thirty-five. Women under the age of thirty-five who had a first-degree relative, mother, sister or father (yes, men do get breast cancer) with breast cancer appeared to have an even greater risk when taking the pill.

Most studies have found no overall increased risk for breast cancer associated with the pill. However, it is difficult to do a meaningful comparison of studies because there have been so many different versions of the pill used by women. The National Women's Health Network has major concerns, warning women that they may be putting themselves at risk by taking oral contraceptives. The network has been pressuring the Food and Drug Administration (FDA) to inform women that long-term use of oral contraceptives might increase the risk of breast cancer and to put that warning on the package inserts.

There is also some evidence that long-term use of the pill may increase the risk of cervical cancer. One study suggested a direct relationship between extended use of the pill, five years or more, and a slightly increased risk. There is some evidence as well that women who never used a barrier method of contraception, such as a diaphragm, or who had a history of genital infections were at higher risk.

The doses of estrogen and progestin in the pill have decreased substantially since the first studies were done, leading Dr. Darcy Spicer, at the University of Southern California, to state, "I think one can fairly conclusively say that oral contraceptives formulated as they are do not increase the risk of breast cancer, presumably because they replace ovarian estrogen and progesterone in amounts which would have been produced by a normal ovary." What's more, Spicer noted preliminary findings in an ongoing clinical trial that suggest that reducing estrogen and progesterone in the pill may be helpful in reducing the risk of breast cancer.

There's other good news as well. Birth control pills may decrease your risk of getting uterine cancer. Women who used a combination pill containing both estrogen and progestin for at least a year have only half the risk of uterine cancer as women who use other types of birth control pills or no oral contraceptives at all. The longer the combination pill is taken, the more the protection increases. In addition, when women went off the pill, the benefits appeared to continue for at least fifteen years.

Women who use the pill are also less likely to get ovarian cancer. A CDC study found that the longer a woman used the pill, the lower her risk was of developing ovarian cancer. Authors of the report estimate that more than 1,700 cases of ovarian cancer in the United States are averted each year by use of the pill. It appears that even women with a family history of ovarian cancer are positively affected by using the pill and that the protection is long-lasting. A possible explanation for that is that the pill creates hormone levels in the body that are similar to those during pregnancy.

༄ ***What to do.*** Stay abreast (no pun intended) of the latest information and discuss the pros and cons with your doctor. Know what pill you are taking, and if it's not a combination pill, containing both estrogen and progestin, ask your doctor why.

༄ *Ovulation*

This is a risk factor over which most of us have no control. Many years ago our ancestors had only about fifty menstrual cycles during a lifetime. Women started menstruating later in life and spent more time pregnant and breast-feeding. Today, the average woman in the United States has about four hundred menstrual cycles, putting her at a greater risk for ovarian, breast, and endometrial cancer.

✍ *What to do.*   Take advantage of screening options.

| ✍ *p53 Gene*

W hen this gene is defective, it may put you at a greater risk of lung cancer. It appears to be defective in virtually every person with the type of lung cancer known as small cell (which accounts for 25 percent of all the lung cancer cases and is the most aggressive) and in half the people with the other type of lung cancer, known as nonsmall cell or large cell. When p53 is normal, it functions as a tumor suppressor gene, one of the body's own natural defenses against cancer. When it is defective, its policing effect is compromised, allowing lung cancer to develop, primarily when the lungs have been damaged by environmental factors, such as smoking. It also may be associated with cancers of the breast, bladder, liver, melanoma, and leukemia.

✍ *What to do.*   Since you can't fix p53 if it is defective, and you may have no way to find out if it is, anyway, decrease any opportunity p53 may have to harm you by limiting, to as great an extent as possible, your exposure to environmental toxins. DON'T SMOKE.

ಐ *Paget's Disease*

I n this condition there is an abnormal development of new bone cells resulting in a larger bone that is weaker and has more blood vessels than normal. Paget's disease is rare and usually affects people over the age of forty. Because osteosarcoma (a form of bone cancer), which is also rare, is most often found in people who have Paget's disease, it is thought by some scientists that osteosarcoma may be triggered by overactivity of bone cells.

ಐ **What to do.** If you have Paget's disease, your condition should be monitored by your doctor.

ಐ *Pap Test (Pap smear)*

T his simple, relatively painless screening test is for cervical cancer. In the last thirty years, the incidence of cervical cancer has risen 3 to 4 percent each year. The mortality rate has dropped a dramatic 70 percent because of the widespread use of the Pap test. This rate could drop even more. Scientists say that most of the cervical cancer deaths could be avoided if all women got regular Pap tests. Because of the long length of time it can take precancerous cells in the cervix to become cancerous, cervical cancer is considered preventable. It is also highly curable when found early.

The Pap test involves scraping some cells from the cervix for examination in order to detect any abnormal, precancerous or malignant cells. The test can also show the presence of infection or inflammation. One way of reporting the results of the Pap test is by the following classes:

- Class 1—There are no abnormal cells.
- Class 2—There are some abnormal cells, but none suggest cancer.
- Class 3—Dysplasia (abnormal growth of cells) is present.
- Class 4—Carcinoma in situ is found.
- Class 5—Invasive cancer is found.

In 1988 a new way of reporting the results of the Pap test was introduced. The Bethesda system is more ambitious and much more complex than the class system. It provides the physician with far more information. It also evaluates the smear sample itself, thereby reducing the likelihood of a false-negative result due to an insufficient sample of cells.

The American Cancer Society and other organizations recommend that you get a Pap test annually when you become sexually active or starting at age eighteen (whichever comes first).

℘ *What to do.*   You can protect yourself from cervical cancer by getting a regular Pap test. It is generally a standard part of a gynecological exam. If you do not go to a gynecologist, go to a facility where you can get a Pap test. It is relatively painless, not time consuming, and inexpensive. It could save your life.

ᆍ *Pelvic Exam*

This is the exam in which the doctor inserts one or two gloved and lubricated fingers into the vagina while placing the other hand on the abdomen to check the vagina, vulva, cervix, fallopian tubes, ovaries, and uterus. It is a major part of a gynecological exam and includes a digital rectal exam. The doctor can get a lot of important information from this exam, including signs of cancer.

ᆍ **What to do.**   You should be having a regular pelvic exam.

ᆍ *Pesticides in Foods*

"We don't believe they pose an unreasonable risk." That's what Environmental Protection Agency (EPA) spokesman Al Heier says about the millions of pounds of pesticides currently being used on farms in the United States. However, according to a report from the National Academy of Sciences, pesticides in foods might be responsible for as many as twenty thousand cancer deaths a year.

The pesticides are usually sprayed directly on crops. They are used to protect crops from insects and crop disease, and kill weeds. Many of the pesticides that contain chemicals that are known to be carcinogenic have not been adequately tested for their health effects on humans—including cancer.

You may recall the Alar controversy in the mid-1980s,

when the phrase "An apple a day . . ." took on a whole new meaning. Alar, which is the trade name for daminozide, had been used for over twenty years on foods from cherries to prunes, but most often on apples. Alar is used to regulate the growth of fruits so that they don't fall from the tree until they're ready. This helps the farmers grow fruits that are cosmetically more attractive and saleable. Alar penetrates the skin of the fruit, and it cannot be washed off. Here's the rub. Since the 1970s Alar has been linked with cancer in various animal studies. In 1985 the EPA proposed a ban on Alar, then decided the evidence was not conclusive and instead placed some restrictions on its use. It ordered the manufacturers to do more safety studies and required a 50 percent reduction in the amount used by farmers. As of February 1990, the use of Alar on foods was totally banned by the EPA.

Another pesticide taken off the market is ethylene dibromide (EDB). This highly successful insect killer was banned by the FDA in 1984 after many studies showed that it caused cancer and genetic mutations in animals.

❧ **What to do.** There are some simple steps you can take to reduce the amount of pesticides to which you are exposed.

LIMITING EXPOSURE TO PESTICIDES ON FOODS

- Wash all fruits and vegetables thoroughly. You may first submerge the vegetables in water with a small amount of a mild detergent to remove pesticides that are nonwatersoluble. Then rinse vigorously with clear water. *Do not soak* the fruits and vegetables—that can remove nutrients.

- Peel fruits and vegetables. With vegetables such as lettuce, cabbage, and brussels sprouts, remove the outer leaves.
- Wash citrus fruits as well. Although generally the amount of pesticides that get through the skin onto the fruit you will eat is so small it should not be a problem, for extra insurance wash the skin. Because it is thought that skins like that of an orange or lemon will not be eaten, a greater amount of pesticide may be used.
- Eat a variety of different fruits and vegetables, so that you decrease your chances of getting a large amount of exposure from one particular food.
- Be extra cautious with exotic, imported fruits, which may contain more pesticides, including ones banned in the United States, like DDT. Again, the key word is *moderation.*
- Although they may look much more appealing, do not buy fruits that have a shiny, waxed coating, because it is not clear that the paraffin is not carcinogenic itself.
- Buy organic produce.
- Ask your supermarket to carry organically grown food.
- Encourage local farmers to reduce their use of pesticides.
- And, although this may not be a practical solution for most people, grow your own fruits and vegetables when you can.

The benefits of a diet rich in fruits and vegetables outweigh the risks of the pesticides they may contain. It is easy to reduce or eliminate the small risk caused by pesticides. Taking the aforementioned simple steps is just one more small component in making your environment as risk free as possible. If you have a question about pesticides, call the EPA pesticide hot line at (800) 858–PEST.

ஜ *Phytochemicals*

These are chemicals found in plants that protect the plants. They also appear to protect people. Various phytochemicals can block the multiple processes that lead to cancer. Although research into phytochemicals is in its infancy, scientists have already identified a number of different phytochemicals that they think may be beneficial in preventing or fighting cancer. A phytochemical in broccoli called sulforaphane appears to prevent breast cancer from developing in lab animals. Dr. Paul Talalay of Johns Hopkins Medical Institute in Baltimore added sulforaphane to human cells in a lab dish and found that it boosted the production of anticancer enzymes. Besides being in broccoli, sulforaphane is present in cauliflower, brussels sprouts, turnips, and kale. Scientists at Cornell University report that of the estimated ten thousand phytochemicals in tomatoes, two of them, p-coumaric acid and chlorogenic acid, activate enzymes that neutralize cancer-causing substances. Those two compounds are found in many fruits and vegetables, including green peppers, pineapples, strawberries, and carrots. Another phytochemical, phenethyl isothiocyanate (PEITC) can be found in vegetables like cabbage. PEITC has been found to inhibit chemical-induced lung cancer in mice and rats. Soybeans contain a phytochemical called genistein. Genistein appears to keep tiny tumors from growing bigger by preventing them from getting the nutrients they

Sources of Phytochemicals

FOOD	HELPFUL SUBSTANCE
Broccoli	*Dithiolthiones*—may block carcinogens from damaging a cell's DNA.
Citrus Fruits	*Limonene*—boosts production of enzymes that might help dispose of potential carcinogens.
Cruciferous Vegetables	*Indoles*—may decrease estrogen in the body, thereby reducing the risk of breast cancer.
	Isothiocyanates—may block carcinogens from damaging a cell's DNA.
Fruits	*Caffeic Acid*—may make carcinogens more soluble in water, which may make it easier to get them out of the body.
	Ferulic Acid—may prevent nitrates from being converted into the carcinogenic nitrosamines.
Garlic, Onions, Leeks, and Chives	*Allyl Sulfides*—may make carcinogens easier to excrete.
	Allium Compounds—may decrease reproduction of tumor cells.
Grains	*Phytic Acid*—may prevent iron from creating cancer-causing free radicals.
Grapes	*Ellagic Acid*—may prevent carcinogens from altering a cell's DNA.

FOOD	HELPFUL SUBSTANCE
Soybeans and Dried Beans	*Protease inhibitors*—may slow tumor growth.
	Phytosterols—may prevent colon cancer by slowing down the reproduction of cells in the large intestine.
	Isoflavones—blocks estrogen's entry into cells, which may reduce the risk of breast and ovarian cancer.
	Saponins—may prevent cancer cells from multiplying.

Source: David Schardt, "Phytochemicals: Plants Against Cancer," *Nutrition Action* (April 1994)

need, by blocking the blood lines that carry oxygen and nutrients. Indole-3-carbinol, a phytochemical found in cauliflower and its relatives, triggers enzymes that break down estrogen, so that it is no longer harmful in promoting breast cancer. And onion and garlic contain allylic sulfide, which can detoxify carcinogens.

🦋 **What to do.**   Include foods that are rich in phytochemicals in your diet.

🦋 Polynuclear Aromatic Hydrocarbons (PAHs)
see "Cooking Carcinogens."

✣ *Polyps*

I t is not uncommon for polyps, small benign growths, to be found in the intestine. Those that are classified as adenomas may become cancerous, particularly if they grow larger than an inch in diameter. Adenomas account for more than 60 percent of all colorectal polyps removed as part of a colonoscopic examination. About 85 percent of adenomas are tubular (growing in tubelike patterns). About 5 percent of adenomas are villious (forming fingerlike projections). The other 10 percent are tubulovillous (a combination of both). Invasive cancer develops in about 5 percent of tubular adenomas, in about 40 percent of villous adenomas, and in about 22 percent of tubulovillous adenomas.

✣ **What to do.** Follow the guidelines for colorectal screening.

✣ *Pregnancy*

I n addition to providing you with another dependent on your income tax, having children can reduce your risk of getting cancer. If you have never been pregnant, or had your first pregnancy after the age of thirty, your risk of developing ovarian and breast cancer is increased. Never having a child increases your risk of endometrial cancer as well. Many studies have established that early full-term pregnancy decreases the risk of breast cancer. However, it appears that the actual benefit may occur only when the woman is older. Studies in Italy and England have indicated a temporary increase in the risk of breast cancer after pregnancy. A large Swedish study found that having a child may increase the risk of breast cancer in younger women (when the incidence of breast cancer is rare), while reducing the risk as the woman gets older, when breast cancer is more common. For the first fifteen years after giving birth, the mother's risk of breast cancer was found to be greater than for women who had not had a child. The older a woman is when she has her first child, the higher her risk of breast cancer right after giving birth. For example, a woman who had her first child at age thirty-five faces a 41 percent higher risk of breast cancer than does a childless woman. But by age fifty-nine, the mother's risk is 29 percent lower than that faced by the childless woman. The risk is lowest in those who give birth at age twenty. By the time they're thirty, the risk of the women in this group is just 2 percent higher than that of a childless woman, and at age fifty-nine it is 32 percent lower. Researchers suggest that a woman's risk of breast cancer may rise for a period of time after giving birth due to stimulation of cells that were already in the early stages of cancer.

It is really not known why pregnancy lowers the risk of breast cancer. The most popular theory to date has been that an early pregnancy would result in a change in hormone levels, most likely in the levels of estrogen. However, according to Dr. Dimitri Trichopoulos, chairman of the department of epidemiology at the Harvard School of Public Health, that is not the case. He says a consensus is gradually emerging that the protective effect of early pregnancy is through differentiation (maturation) of mammary gland cells, which ultimately reduces the number of cells in the breast that are susceptible to cancer. Decreasing the number of cells at risk in the cellular population decreases the number of possible cells that can become cancerous.

Malcolm Pike, M.D., at the University of Southern California, theorizes that early pregnancy transforms breast cells so that fewer are susceptible to harmful effects of estrogen. Therefore, the earlier you go through pregnancy, the earlier this protection kicks in.

Yet another theory is that breast cancer is promoted by the monthly bombardment of breast tissue by hormones, which has its greatest effect on immature, or undifferentiated, breast cells. Pregnancy pushes breast cells to mature (differentiate) and gives breast tissue a nine-month break from the hormonal bombardment.

✤ **What to do.** Getting pregnant and having a child to reduce your risk of getting cancer is obviously not a practical option. But being aware that your risk may be slightly increased if you had your first child after the age of thirty or have never had children should alert you to the importance of doing all the things that you can do to reduce other risks—as well as taking the necessary steps to detect cancer as early as possible, when it is most curable.

✤ *Prophylactic Mastectomy*

"Prophylactic mastectomy may possibly be the most effective intervention we have at the present time to prevent breast cancer." That statement is from Dr. Kelman Cohen, Medical College of Virginia in Richmond, in 1993. Prophylactic mastectomy is also the most radical and extreme intervention. But having your breasts removed is a way to virtually eliminate your risk of breast cancer. Some women at particularly high risk of breast cancer do decide to have a prophylactic mastectomy before there are any signs of cancer. Prophylactic mastectomies reduce the risk by nearly 100 percent, and it would be highly unlikely that a woman who had undergone the operation would get breast cancer. But even when the breasts are removed, there is always the possibility of some minuscule amount of breast tissue remaining, in which breast cancer could develop. That is why it's impossible to offer a guarantee that, even if you take the most extreme prevention measures, you will not get breast cancer.

Cohen, who is chief of plastic surgery at the Medical College of Virginia, says that one of his patients who underwent a prophylactic mastectomy developed breast cancer afterward, and that he knows of several other women who have had the same experience. For that reason, he says that it may be possible that "less tissue is actually a target for breast cancer."

Someone who has been an eyewitness to, and even a participant in, the overenthusiasm for prophylactic mastectomy is John R. Jarrett, M.D., a plastic and reconstructive surgeon in Eugene, Oregon. During the 1970s and 1980s, Jarrett performed some five hundred prophylactic mastectomies on healthy women. He says, "There are a lot of things that we know now that we didn't know in the late seventies" and that had he been going by the standards of 1993, he probably would have performed only half that number (which still sounds like a lot to many people). He notes that today we have improved mammographic techniques and greater knowledge and understanding of benign conditions.

Marc Lippman, M.D., director of the Vincent Lombardi Center at Georgetown University, says about a dozen prophylactic mastectomies are done each year at the center. He advises any woman who is considering this procedure to be aware of all her options before making a decision. He does believe there are some rare situations in which prophylactic mastectomy may be the best solution.

Mary Jo Kahn was diagnosed with breast cancer at the age of thirty-nine. She and her sisters had seen their mother die of breast cancer at the age of forty-seven, after being diagnosed with the disease at the age of thirty-nine. "It was traumatic for all of us," she says. "We felt emotionally orphaned when she died. . . . We all knew we were at risk. While I was in the hospital, my older sister was diagnosed with breast cancer. While we were on chemo, my younger sister and her husband came up. They were adamant that this not happen to her. She checked with many doctors. In the end she had five doctors with whom she conferred. None said to do [a prophylactic mastectomy]. They said it was a viable option. In the end, when she decided to do the prophylactic mastectomy, she went to a surgeon who said, 'I would have never told you to do it, but I'm delighted you're doing it.' The mammograms for my other younger sister were impossible to read. After she had her second biopsy she started looking into prophylactic mastectomy. She had it when she was thirty-three. She was tired of biopsies. Both sisters are happy with it."

There are some doctors who advocate prophylactic

mastectomy for any woman with two immediate family members diagnosed with breast cancer before menopause, but both critics and supporters agree that prophylactic mastectomy is a very radical option to prevent the development of breast cancer.

Most physicians are reluctant to recommend it and do not like to perform it. Susan Love, who is one of those physicians, acknowledges that she has performed a few prophylactic mastectomies in her practice, but only after much time was spent with each woman, going over her breast-cancer risk and the other options open to her, such as very close observation. Love is concerned that this is not always the approach and that there may be women undergoing this procedure unnecessarily. She says, "I think a lot of times women are being sold a bill of goods, and that worries me." Love adds that there have been no studies, and consequently no data, to show that the procedure really does reduce risk. She acknowledges that intuitively it makes sense, but says "a lot of things in medicine that are later proven wrong or harmful, like DES [diethylstilbestrol, the drug given to prevent miscarriage and later found to cause cancer], made sense at the time."

№ *What to do.* Discuss your options with your doctor. You may also want to go for genetic counseling to find out just how much at risk you really are. To find a genetics counselor near you, ask your doctor or call the National Cancer Institute's Cancer Information Service at (800) 4–CANCER. (See "Heredity.")

‿ *Prophylactic Oophorectomy*

To reduce the risk of developing ovarian cancer, some women with a family history of this disease opt to have their ovaries removed. However, there is no clear data on the efficacy of this.

‿ **What to do.** This is an extreme solution, which should be discussed with your doctor. You may also want to speak with a genetics counselor to assess your risk as accurately as possible. To find a genetics counselor near you, ask your doctor or call the National Cancer Institute's Cancer Information Service at (800) 4–CANCER. (See "Heredity.")

‿ *Psychological Factors*

When I had a recurrence of breast cancer, I at first felt that I was responsible for it, that I had brought it on myself. I had suffered some losses and was under a fair amount of stress. Blaming myself and feeling guilty only increased the burden. It was a great relief when I came to the conclusion that I was not responsible for the cancer coming back, that it was not my fault. I certainly knew many people who were under far more stress than I was and who had not gotten cancer.

In recent years there has been tremendous controversy over the role that psychological factors, such as emotions, depression, and stress, play in cancer. This is not something new. The Greek physician Galen, who was born around 130 A.D., observed that melancholy women developed breast cancer more often than other women. In the mid-nineteenth century, British surgeon Sir James Paget wrote that the growth or increase of cancer was influenced by deep anxiety, deferred hope, disappointment, and depression. In 1885, when President Ulysses Grant died of cancer at the age of sixty-three, a neurologist named C. H. Hughes contended that Grant's cancer had been a result of a "wounded spirit." The Civil War hero had seen his reputation ruined by his scandal-ridden second administration.

The mind-body connection movement picked up in the middle of this century. One of its leaders was the research psychologist, Dr. Lawrence LeShan, who studied the role of personality and emotions in the development of cancer. In 1959, after interviewing over 250 cancer patients and comparing them with healthy men and women, his findings were published in the *Journal of the National Cancer Institute.* In his study, 77 percent of the cancer patients had lost a major relationship (parent, child, spouse) before being diagnosed with cancer while only 14 percent of the healthy control group had experienced such a loss; 64 percent couldn't express hostility compared to 32 percent of the control group; 79 percent had feelings of disliking and distrusting themselves, while 34 percent of the controls expressed those feelings; and 38 percent of the cancer patients felt tension from their relationship with one or both parents compared with 12 percent of the control group. But Jimmie Holland, M.D., chief of psychiatry at Memorial Sloan-Kettering Cancer Center, points out it is not known what other factors may or may not have played a role, such as smoking, drinking, etc. She does not support the thesis that one causes one's own cancer or that with enough deter-

mination and positive thinking, one can be cured. But
she does say that there is evidence that the body's physi-
ology may be altered by the intense anxiety experienced
by some patients at high risk of getting cancer, such as
women with close relatives who have died of breast cancer. The theory is that stress or anxiety or depression can
take a toll on the immune system, giving cancer cells a
better environment in which to proliferate. The question
is, do extreme emotions cause a person's immune system
to be lowered or do they cause a person to indulge in
unhealthy practices, such as smoking, drinking alcohol,
overeating, or not eating?

Studies in different countries have come up with findings that people with more social ties and support have a
lower mortality rate from cancer. Is that because they
had better health habits and got better medical care, or
was there some kind of physiological effect from feeling
cared about?

Dr. David Spiegel, at the Stanford Medical School in
California, says, "It is known that psychosocial support
can affect the way patients and their family adjust to their
illness." In a study conducted by Spiegel and others, it
was shown that direct confrontation with fears of dying
and death and venting of strong emotion in a supportive
setting is effective in improving patients' and their families' ability to cope with the illness. In a study of eighty-
six women with metastatic breast cancer, one group received standard medical care, while the other group had
the same care along with a year of weekly one-and-a-half-
hour sessions of supportive-expressive group therapy.
Patients in the control group, who did not have the group
support, suffered a substantial worsening of their mood,
including feelings of anxiety, depression, fatigue, confu-

sion, and loss of vigor. Patients in the support group had the opposite response, showing an improvement in mood. Spiegel was not particularly surprised by the results. The study confirmed his thinking that even a confrontation with death in the form of a terminal illness could be a period of growth and life enhancement rather than emotional decline. And while that result didn't surprise him, another did, greatly. After four years all the women in the control group had died, while one third of the patients in the support group were still living. The mean survival, from the time of study entry until death, was 18.9 months for the control group and 58.4 months for the intervention group, a significant statistical difference. "We came to the conclusion," says Spiegel, "after three years of reanalysis of the data, that something about the intervention had influenced survival time." However, encouraging as that is, it does not tell us whether having strong emotional support can decrease the risk of developing cancer.

The National Cancer Institute is currently funding a study on the links between psychological stress, the immune system, and the development of cancer.

What to do. There is no concrete evidence that feeling good about yourself and being able to handle anxiety, anger, and depression will keep you from getting cancer or even reduce your risk. On the other hand, if you do feel good about yourself, you will enjoy a much better quality of life, which will unquestionably be more satisfying and productive. Who knows, maybe at the same time you will be reducing your risk of cancer.

| ✌ *Radiation Therapy*

A cure or a killer? Radiation has been used as a treatment for various cancers for many years. More than half the people diagnosed with cancer at some point receive some radiation therapy. But when radiation is killing cancer cells, it is also killing healthy cells and raising the possibility of a new cancer in the future. The chest, thyroid, and bone marrow are particularly sensitive to radiation. Patients who receive radiation treatment for ankylosing spondylitis (a painful condition of the spine) have an increased incidence of leukemia. Some data suggest that 5 to 10 percent of patients treated with chemotherapy and radiation for Hodgkin's disease develop acute leukemia within two to twelve years after their first treatment.

New, sophisticated equipment can target the area to be treated and do minimal damage to healthy tissue. The very small possibility of the development of a secondary cancer must be weighed against the known benefits of treatment.

✌ **What to do.**   Make sure the radiologic equipment at the facility where you are receiving the radiation therapy is up to date and that the radiologist and X-ray technician are certified.

| ✌ *Retinoids*

These are synthetic forms of vitamin A that are being studied for their ability to prevent or reduce the risk of skin and lung cancer.

ৡ **What to do.** If you are really concerned about skin and lung cancer, protect yourself from the sun and DON'T SMOKE.

| ৡ *Saccharin*
see "Artificial Sweeteners."

| ৡ *Screening*

S creening for cancer involves the use of various tests to detect cancer in a person who does not have symptoms. It is classified as secondary prevention. Its goal is to prevent death from a cancer by detecting it as early as possible, when there is the best chance of cure or at least prolonged survival. Unfortunately, screening tests are not available for all cancers. Therefore it behooves us to make use of the tests that are. The cancers to which we, as women, are susceptible that do have screening tests are breast (breast self-exam, clinical breast exam, mammography), cervical (pelvic exam, Pap test), colorectal (digital rectal exam, occult stool blood test, flexible sigmoidoscopy), and skin. See individual entries for the individual tests. The following are very general guidelines for screening, which are subject to change:

BREAST

- Between twenty and forty years of age—monthly breast self-exam; clinical exam of breasts by doctor every three years.

- Between forty and fifty years of age—monthly BSE; yearly clinical exam of breasts by doctor; mammography every one to two years.
- Fifty and older—monthly BSE; yearly clinical exam of breasts by doctor; mammography every year.

CERVIX

- Yearly Pap test and pelvic exam starting at age eighteen or when a woman becomes sexually active, whichever comes first.
- Women exposed to DES before birth—yearly Pap test and pelvic exam starting at age fourteen or the start of menstruation, whichever comes first.
- Women who have had a hysterectomy—pelvic exam and Pap test to check vaginal walls for cancer, discuss with doctor.
- Women with a history of infertility, obesity, failure to ovulate, uterine bleeding, or unopposed estrogen or tamoxifen therapy—an endometrial tissue sample should be taken at menopause and thereafter at the discretion of the doctor.

COLORECTAL

- Every adult after the age of forty—digital rectal exam when seen for a periodic exam.
- Starting at age fifty—sigmoidoscopy every three to five years.
- Starting at age fifty—annual occult blood stool test.

<u>SKIN</u>

- Regular self-examination of your skin.
- Starting at age forty—yearly examination by your dermatologist.

&ə **What to do.** If you are not at an increased risk for any of these cancers, follow the guidelines. If you are at a higher risk for a particular cancer, discuss with your doctor whether you would benefit from more frequent screening or more extensive, complex (and frequently costly) tests.

&ə *Secondhand Smoke*
see in "Your Home and Workplace."

&ə *Selenium*

Selenium is an essential mineral that acts as an antioxidant. It can substitute for vitamin E in some of that vitamin's antioxidant activities. An epidemiologic study published in 1995 found no relationship between higher levels of selenium and a reduced risk of cancer in women. The only possible exception appeared to be breast cancer. The authors of the study concluded that their findings provided evidence against the hypothesis that there was an overall protective effect of selenium within the range of selenium ingested in food by women in the United States. However, in an editorial in the same medical journal that published the study, some doctors said the findings should not be the sole basis upon which individual or public health decisions are made, especially since other epidemiologic studies have come up with conflicting results. They called for more studies of the possible role of selenium in reducing the risk of cancer.

SOURCES OF SELENIUM

- brazil nuts
- fish
- foods grown in selenium-rich soil
- kidney
- liver
- muscle meats
- peanuts
- shellfish
- whole-grain cereal

&a *What to do.* Include some selenium-rich foods in your diet. It can't hurt, and it might help. Don't go overboard, though. Too much selenium can cause loss of hair and nails, lesions of the nervous system and skin, and possible damage to your teeth.

&a Sex

Sex . . . a risk factor for cancer? The answer is a qualified yes—but only rarely. Women who delay sexual activity until the age of twenty and who have monogamous relationships reduce their risk of cervical cancer. The risk of developing cervical cancer increases progressively with the number of different partners as well as the number of partners those partners have. (We don't have much control over the number of partners a lover has had!)

What to do. A far greater risk associated with multiple sexual partners is AIDS. So it makes good sense to be cautious and avoid casual sexual encounters.

Sigmoidoscopy (proctosigmoidoscopy)

This test is used as a screening procedure for the early detection of colorectal cancer. A sigmoidoscope—a lighted, tubular instrument—is inserted into the anus. It allows the doctor to see the walls of the rectum and part of the colon, where more than half of all large-bowel cancers occur. This test can be uncomfortable but is usually not painful, lasting about ten minutes. If you are getting a sigmoidoscopy, your doctor will give you instructions to follow before the exam.

What to do. You should have a sigmoidoscopy every three to five years after you turn fifty.

Silicone Implants

Studies have confirmed that silicone breast implants with polyurethane plastic coatings can break down and can send potentially carcinogenic chemicals into women's bodies in small amounts. The research was done by Bristol-Myers Squibb, whose subsidiary Medical Engineering Corporation, made the implants until 1991. Sibyl Goldrich, founder of the Command Trust Network, a consumer information group, wasn't surprised by the finding. "We have known for some time that doctors were not taking seriously enough the issue of polyurethane in our bodies. But the question is, now what? I can't imagine any woman with this cancer-causing stuff coursing through her body just leaving them in place." The FDA says that 2-toluene diamine, or TDA, was found in the blood and urine of women who have the implants. TDA has caused cancer in rats when fed to them. In 1991 the FDA suggested that the risk was so small that removing the implants might pose a bigger risk than leaving them in place.

That same year, implants without the polyurethane coating were scrutinized as well, because of concern that the silicone in the implants might also cause health problems, such as immune system breakdowns. The FDA requested the removal of all silicone gel implants from the market.

What to do. Although it is unlikely that silicone breast implants will cause cancer, if you have them you may want to discuss it with your doctor and be sure that you do all the things you can to detect breast cancer early as well to reduce your risk of developing it.

ᥓᥩ Skin Self-exam

This is a simple screening you can do to find signs of skin cancer—melanoma or nonmelanoma—as early as possible. A skin self-exam is easy to do, free, and does not take very long. The best time to do this is after a shower or bath in a well-lit room with a full-length mirror. A hand-held mirror is also helpful. It's best to begin by learning where your birthmarks, moles, and blemishes are and what they look and feel like. That way you'll be able to tell if there are any changes. Check for anything new: you're looking for a change in the size, texture, shape, consistency, or color of a mole, or for a sore that does not heal. Check all areas of your body, including the back, scalp, between the buttocks, and the genital area.

DOING A SKIN SELF-EXAM

Step 1. Look at the front and back of your body in the mirror, then raise your arms and look at your left and right sides.

Step 2. Bend your elbows and look carefully at your palms, forearms, including the undersides, and upper arms.

Step 3. Examine the back and front of your legs. Also look between the buttocks and around the genital area.

Step 4. Sit and closely examine your feet, including the soles and the spaces between the toes.

Step 5. Look at your face, neck, and scalp. You may want to use a comb or blow dryer to move hair so that you can see better.

✍ **What to do.**   If you find anything unusual, see your doctor right away. The earlier skin cancer is found, the better the chance for a cure.

✍ *Smoking*

No buts about it, cigarette smoking is responsible for about 30 percent of all cancer deaths in the United States every year. It is the most important, significant carcinogenic hazard in the United States. Forty-three carcinogens have been identified in tobacco smoke. As many as 90 percent of all cases of lung cancer are found in people who smoke. Smoking is also linked to cancers of the larynx, mouth, pharynx, esophagus, bladder (it's a contributing factor in up to a third of the women with bladder cancer), and pancreas; recent evidence also indicates a link between smoking and cancers of the kidney (possibly causing more than 25 percent of the cases), pelvis, cervix, nasal passages, stomach, breast, and leukemia.

In 1964 the U.S. Surgeon General's first report on the health risks of cigarette smoking was released. It contained strong evidence of the association between smoking and cancer. Since that time the evidence has been accumulating. In 1987 lung cancer took over as the leading cause of cancer death in women. Before that, breast cancer had held that dubious distinction. The incidence for lung cancer in women continues to increase, while the incidence is decreasing for men.

The younger you are when you start smoking, the more you smoke each day, and the longer you've been smoking, all increase your risk of developing lung and other smoking-associated cancers. When you quit, your risk of lung and other cancers begins to decrease and continues to decline gradually each year. After fifteen to twenty years, the ex-smoker's risk of dying of lung cancer may approach that of someone who has never smoked.

If you have breast cancer and smoke, you are at an at least 25 percent increased risk of dying from breast cancer. According to an ACS study, reported in June 1994, the risk grows with the number of cigarettes a woman smokes. Women smoking two or more packs a day have an escalated risk of dying from breast cancer compared to nonsmokers and former smokers. Eugenia Calle, the epidemiologist who directed the study, said the findings did not suggest that smoking causes breast cancer. She said there were several possibilities for the increased mortality risk, which include the facts that "smokers may have impaired immune systems, they may not obtain routine [mammograms], or smoking may cause a direct deleterious effect on survival."

Cigarette by-products can be deposited in gynecologic tissue. It is thought that a high level of nicotine in the cervical mucosa can compromise the immune system in the cervix, making it more susceptible to viral infection, such as human papillomavirus, a risk factor for cervical cancer.

If you smoke, quitting could be the smartest health move you could ever make. It is not easy to quit. Anyone who tells you it is, is lying. Smoking is more than just a habit, it's a physical addiction. But difficult as it is, many people do quit, and you really should, too, if you do smoke.

TIPS TO QUIT SMOKING

Getting Ready

- Make the decision to quit and acknowledge that it will be difficult and *not* enjoyable. Make a list of your reasons for stopping.
- Decide how you will quit: cold turkey (choosing a date and just stopping), or gradually decreasing the amount of cigarettes you smoke each day.
- Notice when and why you smoke. What are the things that make you want to have a cigarette?
- Change your smoking routines: keep your cigarettes in a different place; change brands; smoke with your other hand; buy one pack at a time.
- Smoke only in certain places, such as outdoors.
- When you want a cigarette, wait one minute and try to think of something else to do instead, such as having a glass of water or going for a stroll.
- Set a date for quitting. If possible, get a friend to quit with you.

The Day Arrives

- Change your morning routine. When you eat breakfast, don't sit in the same place. If you always drink coffee, switch to tea.
- Get rid of any cigarettes you have left. Wet them, so that even if you want to retrieve them, you will not be able to smoke them. Put away, or throw away, your ashtrays.
- Carry other things around to put in your mouth such as gum, hard candy, or a toothpick.
- At the end of the day give yourself a reward for not

smoking—maybe a movie you've been wanting to see or your favorite meal.

- Start a money jar (my favorite). Each day put in the money you saved by not smoking.

Staying Quit . . .

- Don't worry if you are sleepier or more short-tempered than usual; that will pass.
- Let other people know that you have quit smoking and that as a result you may be a little irritable. Most people will support you. Some of your smoking friends may even ask for advice on how to quit.
- Exercise. Take walks or bike rides. Join a gym.
- Keep the list you made of your reasons for quitting with you and when you get a craving for a cigarette, go over all the positive things about not smoking.
- When you feel tense, try to keep busy, think about ways to solve the problem, tell yourself that smoking won't make it any better, and go do something else.
- Eat regular meals. Feeling hungry is sometimes mistaken for the desire to smoke.
- If you slip and smoke, don't be discouraged and don't beat up on yourself. Many smokers try to quit several times before they quit for good. Quit again.

If you need more help, see your doctor. She may prescribe nicotine gum or a nicotine patch to help you break your addiction to cigarettes. The American Cancer Society and the Lung Association run smoking-cessation programs. (Their addresses and telephone numbers are in the appendix.) Call the National Cancer Institute's toll-free Cancer Information Service at (800) 4–CANCER for free publications on quitting, as well as information on smoking-cessation programs in your area.

ℰ **What to do.** QUIT.

| ℰ *Soy*

S oybeans and soybean products, like tofu, tempeh, miso, and soy milk, appear to be tied to a lower risk of many cancers, including breast and colon cancer. Soybeans are an especially rich source of isoflavones. Isoflavones are potent phytochemicals that are thought to be responsible for lowering the risk of ovarian and breast cancer by blocking the entry of estrogen into cells. In 1963 scientists in Germany isolated a phytochemical in soybeans that can block capillaries that bring oxygen and other nutrients to tumors. This chemical is called genistein.

To get the effects of soy products, you need just two ounces a day of soy protein. You can get that in one half of a cup of tofu, one third of a cup of soy flour, or one cup of soy milk. You should be able to find tofu in the fresh produce section of your supermarket. It comes in several forms: firm, extra firm, soft, and silken. It is rich in isoflavones, relatively low in saturated fat, low in sodium, and cholesterol free.

OTHER SOY PRODUCTS

- Tempeh is a dense, chewy, textured soyfood with a nutty, slightly smoky taste. It is a good source of isoflavones, fiber, protein, and vitamin B.

- Miso, a fermented soybean paste, is widely used in Japan to flavor soups and salad dressings and as a condiment. It is a good source of protein, isoflavones, and antioxidant compounds. It is low in fat but has a high salt content.
- Soy milk is liquid made from ground whole soybeans and water. It is a good source of protein, isoflavones, B vitamins, and minerals. It can be used for drinking or as a complete milk replacement in recipes.
- Textured soy protein is made from compressed soy flour. It is a good source of isoflavones and calcium.

๛ **What to do.**   Include soy products in your diet. For recipes and information call the United Soybean Hotline at (800) TALK SOY.

๛ Spray Cans
see "Aerosols."

๛ Squamous Intraepithelial Lesion (SIL) (dysplasia; cervical intraepithelial neoplasia [CIN])
see "Cervical Dysplasia."

✌ Stool Guaiac Test
see "Occult Blood Stool Test."

✌ Stress
see "Psychological Factors."

✌ Sugar
see "Artificial Sweeteners."

✌ Talcum Powder

S ome researchers theorize that the use of talcum powder in the anal and vaginal area might increase the risk of ovarian cancer. The reasoning is that the talcum powder can enter the reproductive tract and settle on the ovary and possibly irritate it, leading to the development of cancer.

✌ **What to do.** If you have any concerns, limit your use of talcum powder or stop using it altogether.

❧ *Tamoxifen (Nolvadex)*

Tamoxifen is an artificial anti-estrogen drug used to treat some women with breast cancer. Can it do more? In April 1992 the Breast Cancer Prevention Trial (BCPT) was started to evaluate whether tamoxifen can also prevent the development of new breast cancers. The trial, which is ongoing, has generated tremendous controversy.

Dr. Bernadine Healy, then head of the National Institutes of Health, called the study "precedent setting," citing estimates that tamoxifen could reduce the incidence of breast cancer in women at risk [over age fifty, family history, and so on] by 30 to 50 percent. Tamoxifen also appears to have other advantages. Studies done by Richard Love at the University of Wisconsin, showed that tamoxifen treatment for breast cancer increased bone density in 140 women by 3 percent. Although that is less than the 5 to 10 percent increase seen in studies using estrogen, it is the same as the anti-osteoporosis drug etidronate.

It sounds too good to be true. Many think it is. At a congressional hearing, Adrian Fugh-Berman, M.D., medical advisor to the Women's Health Network, said that "the women eligible for enrollment [in BCPT] are not truly at high risk for breast cancer, and tamoxifen is too toxic for use in healthy women. . . . While the benefits of tamoxifen for primary prevention are highly questionable, the risks are well-documented." More criticism came from Samuel Epstein, M.D., professor of occupational and environmental health at the University of Illinois at the Medical Center in Chicago. He says that there is not "the slightest scrap of evidence that tamoxifen will prevent breast cancer. It is a powerful liver carcinogen and also produces cancer of the uterus." In March 1994 new data emerged suggesting that tamoxifen may be riskier than previously thought. It appeared to have the potential of causing fatal uterine cancer.

Experts assured the women with breast cancer who were being treated with tamoxifen that the drug's proven benefit in preventing new breast cancers outweighed its risks and that the debate was only about healthy women taking the drug in the BCPT. NCI contended that tamoxifen could conceivably prevent 133 cases of cancer while causing 83 cases of uterine cancer. Critics continued to say that tamoxifen could do far more harm.

℘ *What to do.* This is a tricky one. The only women eligible for BCPT are those who are considered at an increased risk of developing breast cancer. If you are in that group and are considering taking part, discuss it with your doctor. You may also want to see a genetics counselor to assess just what your risk is before making a decision.

℘ *Vegetables*

In your diet of at least five fruits and vegetables a day, you should have more vegetables than fruits. The following chart is a simple way to see quickly which vegetables provide the greatest source of vitamin A, vitamin C, vitamin E, calcium, fiber, folic acid (or folate), and copper:

Benefits

VEGETABLE	AMT	A	C	E	CALCIUM	FIBER	FOLIC ACID (OR FOLATE)	COPPER
artichoke	1 med		*			*	*	
asparagus	1/2 cup		**				*	
beans	1/2 cup		*			*		*
bean sprouts	1/2 cup		*					
beets	1/2 cup					*	*	
broccoli	1/2 cup	*	**		*	*	*	
brussels sprouts	1/2 cup		**			*	*	
cabbage	1/2 cup		**			*		
carrots	1/2 cup	**				*		
cauliflower	1/2 cup		**				*	
chards	1/2 cup	**	*	*				
Chinese cabbage	1/2 cup		**					*
collards	1/2 cup	*	*					
corn	1/2 cup						*	
dandelion greens	1/2 cup		*	*				
endive, chicory romaine, escarole	1 cup	*					*	
kale	1/2 cup	**	**					
kohlrabi	1/2 cup		**	*				
mustard greens	1/2 cup	*	*	*				
okra	1/2 cup		*			*	*	
onion	1 med		*				*	
parsnips	1/2 cup		*			*	*	
peas	1/2 cup	**	*				*	
pepper	1 small	**	**					
plantain	1 med	*						
potato	1 med		*			*		*
pumpkin	1/2 cup	*	*	*				

VEGETABLE	AMT	A	C	E	CALCIUM	FIBER	FOLIC ACID (OR FOLATE)	COPPER
radishes	6 large		*					
rutabagas	1/2 cup		*					
snow peas	1/2 cup		**			*		
spinach	1/2 cup	**	*	*		*	*	
squash	1/2 cup		*			*		
sweet potato	1 med	**	**			*		*
tomatoes	1 med	*	*			*		*
turnip greens	1/2 cup	**	*	*	*		*	*
watercress	1/2 cup		*					

**especially good source

🌿 ***What to do.*** Eat those veggies. Raw vegetables make excellent healthy snacks. They are often available at your supermarket already cut and cleaned. Although having someone else prepare them may add to the cost of the vegetables, buying them cleaned and cut is definitely worth considering if you are low on time and money is not a problem. Use fresh or frozen vegetables. If cooking, steam or microwave vegetables to preserve as much nutritional quality and flavor as possible.

🌿 *Vitamin A*

According to a report by researchers at the University of Arizona in Tucson, a synthetic form of vitamin A called all-*trans*-retinoic acid appeared to be capable of reversing early precancerous changes in cervical cells. In 47 percent of the women treated with the retinoic acid, moderate dysplasia was reversed; whereas in women getting a placebo, the reversal occurred in 27 percent of those women. Cervical dysplasia often goes away by itself.

Many laboratory studies on rats have shown and continue to show that retinoids (vitamin A or synthetics of vitamin A) at high doses reduce breast cancer. Adrianne Rogers, M.D., at the department of pathology, Boston University School of Medicine, explains that the doses of vitamin A given the rats were extremely high, as much as three hundred times the requirement (the recommended daily requirement for women is 800 retinol equivalents a day), and that given to humans at that level, vitamin A would be very toxic. But she says there are many studies being done with different synthetic retinoids, in hopes of finding ones that will reduce the risk of breast cancer without toxic effects. The chief obstacle, in terms of long-term use of retinoids for the prevention of breast cancer, is toxicity, as most retinoids accumulate in the liver and can cause liver failure. A relatively nontoxic retinoid called fenretinide has been developed and is being investigated in a long-term clinical trial for its effectiveness in preventing second primary breast tumors.

Clifford Welsch, Ph.D., at the department of pharmacology and toxicology, Michigan State University, says that studies using lower levels of vitamin A had no effect, that near-toxicity levels are required to get an antitumor effect in animals. Welsch calls retinoids a "double-edged sword" because there are studies that show retinoids inhibiting tumor growth and other studies that show retinoids exciting and enhancing the tumor process. In 1992 a study was conducted in which large doses of retinoids were given to human subjects. There were no apparent

Sources of Vitamin A

FOOD	AMOUNT	% OF U.S. RDA
GRAIN PRODUCTS		
fortified cereals	1 oz	25–39
oatmeal	2/3 cup	over 40
FRUIT		
apricot	1/2 cup	25–39
apricot nectar	1/2 cup	10–24
cantaloupe	1/2 cup	25–39
mandarin orange sections	1/2 cup	10–24
mango	1/2 med	over 40
nectarine	1 med	10–24
plums	1/2 cup	10–24
watermelon	1 3/4 cup	10–24
VEGETABLES—COOKED		
broccoli	1/2 cup	10–24
carrots	1/2 cup	over 40
chards	1/2 cup	10–24
collards	1/2 cup	10–24
endive, chicory, romaine, escarole	1 cup	10–24
kale	1/2 cup	over 40
mustard greens	1/2 cup	10–24
peas	1/2 cup	over 40
pepper	1 small	over 40
plantain	1 med	10–24
pumpkin	1/2 cup	10–24
spinach	1/2 cup	over 40
squash	1/2 cup	over 40

FOOD	AMOUNT	% OF U.S. RDA
sweet potato	1 med	over 40
tomatoes	1 med	10–24
turnip greens	½ cup	over 40

Meat, Poultry, Fish

liver		
beef, calf, pork,	2 oz	over 40
chicken, turkey	½ cup diced	over 40
mackerel	3 oz	10–24

Milk

low-fat or skim	1 cup	10–24

Source: U.S. Department of Agriculture.

serious side effects, other than occupational night blindness that was relatively easily reversed.

Vitamin A may offer some protection against lung cancer.

ða **What to do.** Include foods with vitamin A in your diet.

ða *Vitamin C*

It can prevent some tumors in laboratory animals. It may prevent cancer-causing nitrosamines from forming in people's stomachs. Overall, the data is not encouraging. In the Harvard Nurses' Health Study, in which some 89,000 women have been followed since 1980, it was found that women who chose to take at least 750 mg a day of C in supplement form had no lower risk of breast cancer than women who did not take the vitamin. Researchers at Dartmouth Medical School found that giving people who had had at least one polyp removed 1000 mg a day of vitamin C did not reduce the number of new polyps.

🎗 **What to do.** Include foods with vitamin C in your diet.

Sources of Vitamin C

FOOD	AMOUNT	% OF U.S. RDA
GRAINS		
fortified cereals	1 oz	25–39
oatmeal, instant, fortified	²/₃ cup	over 40
FRUITS		
apple juice	³/₄ cup	over 40
cantaloupe	¹/₂ cup	over 40
cranberry juice	1 cup	over 40
grapefruit	¹/₂ med	over 40
grapefruit juice	³/₄ cup	over 40
grape juice, unsweetened	³/₄ cup	over 40
honeydew melon	³/₄ cup	over 40
kiwifruit	1 med	over 40
mandarin orange sections	³/₄ cup	over 40

FOOD	AMOUNT	% OF U.S. RDA
mango	1/2 med	over 40
orange	1 med	over 40
papaya	1/4 med	over 40
peaches	1/2 cup	over 40
pear	1 med	over 40
pineapple/grapefruit juice	3/4 cup	over 40
pineapple juice	3/4 cup	25–39
pineapple/orange juice	3/4 cup	over 40
plum	1 med	10–24
pomegranate	1 med	10–24
raspberries	1/2 cup	25–39
strawberries	1/2 cup	over 40
tangelo	1 med	over 40
tangerine	1 med	over 40
watermelon	1 3/4 cup	over 40

VEGETABLES—COOKED

FOOD	AMOUNT	% OF U.S. RDA
artichoke	1 med	10–24
asparagus	1/2 cup	over 40
beans, green or yellow	1/2 cup	10–24
bean sprouts	1/2 cup	10–24
broccoli	1/2 cup	over 40
brussels sprouts	1/2 cup	over 40
cabbage, red	1/2 cup	over 40
cauliflower	1/2 cup	over 40
chard	1/2 cup	10–24
collards	1/2 cup	10–24
dandelion greens	1/2 cup	10–24
endive (raw)	1 cup	10–24
kale	1/2 cup	over 40
kohlrabi	1/2 cup	over 40
mustard greens	1/2 cup	25–39

FOOD	AMOUNT	% OF U.S. RDA
okra	1/2 cup	10–24
onion	1 large	10–24
parsnips	1/2 cup	10–24
peas	1/2 cup	10–24
pepper, green or red	1/2 cup	over 40
plantain, green or ripe	1 med	over 40
poke greens	1/2 cup	over 40
potato w/skin	1 med	25–39
pumpkin	1/2 cup	10–24
radishes (raw)	6 large	10–24
rutabagas	1/2 cup	25–39
snow peas	1/2 cup	over 40
spinach	1/2 cup	10–24
squash	1/2 cup	10–24
sweet potato		
baked or boiled	1 med	over 40
canned	1/2 cup	over 40
tomatoes	1/2 cup	25–39
tomato juice (canned)	3/4 cup	over 40
turnip greens with turnips	1/2 cup	10–24
watercress (raw)	1/2 cup	10–24

MEAT, FISH

chicken	1/2 cup	10–24
clams, mussels	3 oz	10–24
liver—beef, pork	3 oz	25–39

Source: U.S. Department of Agriculture.

℘ *Vitamin E (alpha tocopherol)*

V itamin E is considered to be the most effective anti-oxidant for getting rid of free radicals in the body. Several studies have suggested that it may play a role in protecting you from cancers of the lung, breast, cervix, stomach, pancreas, and urinary tract. Vitamin E also appears to play a role in building up the immune system, which could enable the body to successfully fight cancer in its earliest stages.

℘ **What to do.**   Include foods rich in vitamin E in your diet.

Sources of Vitamin E

FOOD	AMOUNT	% OF U.S. RDA
GRAIN PRODUCTS		
multigrain cereals, cooked	²/₃ cup	10–24
ready-to-eat cereals, fortified	1 oz	over 40
wheat germ, plain	2 tbs	
VEGETABLES—COOKED		
chard	¹/₂ cup	10–24
dandelion greens	¹/₂ cup	10–24
kohlrabi	¹/₂ cup	10–24
mustard greens	¹/₂ cup	10–24
pumpkin	¹/₂ cup	10–24
turnip greens	¹/₂ cup	10–24

FOOD	AMOUNT	% OF U.S. RDA

FRUITS

apple, baked, unsweetened	1 med	10–24
apricots, canned, juice-pack	½ cup	10–24
nectarine, raw	1 med	10–24
peaches, canned, juice-pack	½ cup	10–24

MEAT, FISH

clams, steamed, boiled or canned, drained	3 oz	10–24
croaker, mackerel, mullet, or ocean perch; baked or broiled	3 oz	10–24
liver, chicken, turkey braised	½ cup diced	10–24
mackerel, canned, drained	3 oz	10–24
salmon, baked, broiled, steamed, or poached	3 oz	10–24
scallops, baked or broiled	3 oz	10–24
shrimp, broiled, steamed, boiled, or canned and drained	3 oz	25–39

NUTS AND SEEDS

almonds, not roasted	2 tbs	over 40
Brazil nuts	2 tbs	10–24
filberts	2 tbs	over 40
peanut butter	2 tbs	25–39
peanuts, roasted or dry-roasted	2 tbs	10–24
sunflower seeds, hulled, roasted, or dry-roasted	2 tbs	over 40

Source: U.S. Department of Agriculture.

ഇ *Water*

Water is a necessity of life. You could go for two
months or longer without food and survive. No
one can survive without water for more than a few days.
So we have to have it. Do we have to be concerned about
it?

Concern over bad water is nothing new. A Sanskrit
manuscript from 2000 B.C. states, "It is good to keep
water in copper vessels, to expose it to sunlight, and filter
it through charcoal." And around 400 B.C. Hippocrates
stressed the importance of water quality to health. He
recommended boiling and straining rainwater.

A survey done by the United States Geological Survey
in 1988 found contamination of groundwater increasing
in every state. In 1995 the Environmental Working
Group tabulated the number of drinking-water complaints made to the Environmental Protection Agency in
1993 and 1994. It found that one in five Americans is
drinking water that violates federal health standards and
that about 25 percent of communities provide water with
excessive levels of biological, chemical, or radioactive
contaminants.

While contaminated water can result in many illnesses, cancer is generally unlikely to be one of them.
However, there are some things to be on the alert for,
regarding your drinking-water supply.

In 1908 water systems in the United States were chlorinated, killing the typhoid and cholera germs, as well as
improving the taste and smell of the water. It was only
later that it was discovered that chlorine could be a hazard. Cancer-causing compounds called total trihalometh-

anes (TTHMs), produced during chlorination, have been found to be carcinogenic and mutagenic in lab tests. A large study found a small risk of bladder cancer associated with prolonged use of chlorinated water. Some researchers estimate that over ten thousand people a year get rectal or bladder cancer caused by chlorinated water. Other researchers say this is a gross overestimate. Today, seven out of ten Americans drink chlorinated water.

Another possible cause of cancer is radioactive contamination of the water. This is generally not from a nearby nuclear power plant but rather the result of radon seeping into groundwater. The long-term effects of drinking water containing radon is not known. Radon in the water plays an insignificant role in the overall levels of radon in the house. If you are concerned about radon in your water, you can have your water tested with a liquid scintillation spectrometer. This must be done by a professional.

Hazardous, possibly carcinogenic, chemicals that may be found in water include benzene, toxaphene, carbon tetrachloride (CTC), p-Dichlorobenzene, 1,2-dichloroethane, trichloroethylene (TCE), TTHM, and vinyl chloride. The sources of these organic chemicals are pesticides, industrial waste products, chlorination, and oil refinery by-products.

Most people in the United States get their water from a public or community system that is federally regulated. In general, the larger the city and the bigger the water supplier, the more likely it is that the water will be healthy, complying with the standards set by the FDA. If you get your water from a well on your property, you, for the most part, are responsible for its quality.

&ᴥ *What to do.* It is not likely that your water contains any of the carcinogenic contaminants, especially if it comes from a public or community system. If it does contain some contaminants, it is extremely unlikely that the levels will pose any hazard to you. However, the only way you'll know for sure is to test the water.

If you have TTHMs in your water, experts recommend letting any water you are going to use sit in an open container for at least six hours to eliminate the chlorine by-products. Cooking also eliminates more of the TTHM's toxicity. Or you can use activated carbon filtration. This involves putting a carbon filter on the faucet or connecting a filter to the pipe that carries water to the faucet. You can also get a filter through which you pour any water you'll be drinking.

If your water has a high level of radon and you want to reduce it, the most common method is installation of a granulated activated carbon (GAC) tank. It should be installed on the incoming water line immediately after the pressure tank. Another way to reduce the radon is by installing an aeration unit in the water line.

For more information call the Safe Drinking Water Hotline at (800) 426–4791, a service of the Environmental Protection Agency.

&ᴥ *X-ray*

X-rays are high-energy radiation that can be used in the diagnosis of cancer and its treatment. In 1895 Wilhelm Roentgen discovered that waves of electromagnetic energy, or "x-rays" as he called them, could penetrate the tissue and enable one to see inside the human body. It was a miraculous discovery. Its use in medicine soon became apparent. When X-rays were first used, the incidence of leukemia among radiologists increased tenfold. Since then, there have been tremendous technological advances in diagnostic X-rays, making them more effective and safe.

As X-ray machines and techniques have improved, the risks associated with diagnostic X-rays have decreased. Possible risks that have been associated with X-rays include leukemia. A study done in Maine on 75,000 people who had had diagnostic X-rays estimated that about 1 percent of leukemia cases and less than 1 percent of breast cancer cases resulted from the diagnostic X-rays. (Only leukemia and breast cancer were looked at.) It is estimated that X-rays may result in a few thousand deaths a year. While that may sound a bit scary, remember that it is less than 1 percent of the 1 million cancers diagnosed in the United States annually.

It is widely felt in the medical field that the benefits greatly outweigh any risk when a diagnostic X-ray is performed for an important medical reason.

What to do. Since X-rays have the potential to be harmful, it is a good idea to get them only when necessary. Whenever your doctor or dentist wants you to have an X-ray, ask why it is necessary, if it will affect diagnosis or treatment, or if it will provide information the doctor does not have. If you are going for a consultation or second opinion, bring your X-rays with you to that doctor, so that additional X-rays do not have to be taken. Keep your own record of what X-rays you've had and when, so that if you are seeing a new doctor, you can tell her what

X-rays you've had in the past. Make sure the radiologic equipment at the facility is up to date and that the radiologist and X-ray technician are certified. When X-rays are done for a good reason, the benefits greatly outweigh the risks.

II

Your Home and Workplace

We think of our home as our safe haven. But is it? Although many women do work outside the home, there are still many women who stay at home with the kids. So some women are likely to have more exposure to hazards in the home than their spouses. There are numerous obvious and not so obvious things in our home that could strike a lethal blow. When people hear the words "air pollution," for example, they usually think of outdoor air, such as smog in Los Angeles. However, indoor air pollution is a far greater hazard. The good news is that virtually all of the hazards in your home that increase your risk of cancer can, with a little effort and in some cases a little money, be eliminated or reduced so they will cause no harm. You cannot change the fact that your mother or sister had breast cancer or that you started menstruating at an early age, but you can change things in your home to make it safe and secure—at least from toxic substances.

The same toxic substances you can encounter in your home can also be present in your workplace: radon, asbestos, secondhand smoke, and electromagnetic fields. Occupational exposures appear to account for about 5 percent of all cancer deaths.

If you are planning to buy a home, there are various hazards that could increase your risk of cancer that you should check for in a house. Once identified, they can usually be successfully eliminated or treated. If you are looking at or building a brand-new home, you also want to be as sure as possible that none of those hazards is

present. There are a number of simple steps you can take
to find and purchase a home that will not put your health
at risk.

- Make as thorough an inspection as possible inside the
  house. Look at every part of the house, carefully. Go
  into the basement. Are there pipes covered with insulation? What is the insulation made of? In what condition is the insulation?
- Outside the house, check the condition of the plant
  life. Does it look healthy? Breathe deeply. Do you notice any suspicious or unexpected odors?
- Ask the owner why is the house being sold, how long
  have they owned it, how old is the house, was asbestos
  ever used for insulation in the house, have they had
  it tested for radon, how is the water, and what is its
  source?
- Check with the local health department to find out if
  there have been any clusters of cancers reported in the
  neighborhood and if there are any known hazardous
  waste sites, and if so, where they are.
- Ask some people in the neighborhood, diplomatically,
  if there have been any "problems" in the area: medical
  problems, water problems, strange odors, and so on.
- In the area, check for any nearby industrial plants or a
  nuclear power plant. If there is a local lake or stream,
  how does the water look (don't taste it!)?
- Check for nearby high-voltage power lines.
- Find out from the real estate agent what the owner is
  obligated, under law, to reveal to you regarding potential hazards in the house.
- If you do not have proof that the house was tested for

radon levels, have a test. If you suspect an asbestos problem, call in a professional.

No matter how much you've fallen in love with a house you want to buy, the affair will be short-lived if once you're living in the house, you discover conditions that make you and your family ill.

৪৯ *Asbestos*

Asbestos is a group of naturally occurring mineral fibers found in rocks. It was widely used in a variety of products and building materials until the late 1970s, when the U.S. Consumer Product Safety Commission banned its use in some products, such as spray-applied insulation, fireproofing, and acoustical surfacing material, that released excessive amounts of asbestos fibers into the environment. Exposure to asbestos has been linked primarily to lung cancer, as well as to cancer of the larynx. Those at the greatest risk are people who work with asbestos. Having it in your home does pose a risk. Your risk of lung cancer increases exponentially if you are exposed to asbestos and also smoke. Before its hazards were known, asbestos was frequently used as insulation in walls in homes and around pipes, boilers, and hot water heaters. It was also used in many different products, including shingles, siding, floor and ceiling tiles, hair dryers, toasters, broilers, refrigerators, and other appliances. If your house was built or remodeled between 1920 and 1970, it may contain asbestos. About one-quarter of those houses do.

Asbestos is only a danger when it is damaged, enabling fibers to escape into the air. You cannot see, feel, or smell those airborne fibers, but you can inhale them. Once you do, they can become lodged in tissue for a long time. There is no way they can be removed. If I've alarmed you—I am sorry. But there is good reason for alarm, asbestos is scary stuff.

If you suspect you may have an asbestos problem in your home, you can do your own preliminary inspection. Remember, asbestos is only a hazard when it is damaged. Look carefully at the condition of any asbestos you find in your home, but don't touch it.

CHECKING FOR ASBESTOS

- Insulation on basement pipes or old boilers and old hot water heaters—look for damage, tears, flaking, or dislodged chunks.
- Installation of asbestos-containing products—if poorly installed, there is a greater possibility of deterioration or damage.
- Water leaks—water can dislodge or disturb the asbestos, and it can dissolve or wash out the material binding the asbestos, increasing the possibility of fibers being released.
- When checking for asbestos, do not touch it to see if it's flaking or coming apart. You should only observe it. There is no known safe level of exposure.

If, in your inspection you find no damage and you feel sure there is not a problem, then just continue to periodically inspect the asbestos. If you think it may be damaged and dangerous, CALL IN AN EXPERT. NEVER try to eliminate asbestos on your own. Get a professional who has been trained in asbestos abatement, if possible someone who is certified or licensed.

FINDING AND ENGAGING A CONTRACTOR

- Call your state asbestos office for a list of certified or approved contractors and for the applicable state regulations regarding its removal.
- Collect evidence of the contractor's experience and/or training in asbestos abatement.
- Obtain and check out their references from previous clients.
- Request a written estimate. It's not a bad idea to get several estimates, as prices can vary, sometimes substantially.
- Find out the specifics of what constitutes successful job completion from your state asbestos office.
- Inquire about their follow-up plans and if they include thorough cleaning of the abatement area, which is absolutely essential, and air monitoring.

There are three ways of dealing with an asbestos problem: removal, enclosure, and encapsulation. Which you choose will depend mainly on the problem's severity. You may use a combination of methods.

WAYS TO ELIMINATE ASBESTOS RISK

- *Removal*—this is the most costly method, but it can solve almost any problem you have. It is a permanent solution, and you will not have to do any maintenance or periodic checks in the future.

- *Enclosure*—this is generally less costly than removal. It involves airtight walls and ceilings being put up around the asbestos. This can be done only if the underlying structure can support new walls and ceilings. Asbestos will continue to be released behind the enclosure, so if the enclosure becomes damaged, in any way, it will require immediate repair. That means you have to carefully check the enclosure regularly.
- *Encapsulation*—this is a method that prevents fibers from being released by applying a sealant. Sealants should be used only on granular, cementlike material and not on materials that are extensively damaged or deteriorated, so it may not be appropriate for your situation. If a sealant is used, regular inspections must be made to make sure it remains intact.

When the job is finished, a thorough cleanup by the contractor is essential. A wet mop is used—*never* a dry mop or broom, because they can cause the fibers to become airborne—on all surfaces. This should be repeated the day after the completion of asbestos treatment or removal to get any suspected fibers that have settled on the floor. Any debris in the surrounding area, along with the clothing worn during the removal, should be put in a 6-millimeter-thick plastic trash bag.

☙ **What to do.** Follow the steps above. Asbestos that is getting into the air is a big risk factor that can and must be eliminated. Although it may take some time and money, do it!

✿ *Electromagnetic Field (EMF)*

E lectromagnetic fields are a combination of electric fields and magnetic fields that radiate from electrical cables, power lines, wires, and fixtures, and electrical appliances, such as refrigerators, freezers, clothes washers, hair dryers, shavers, food mixers, blenders, vacuums, space heaters, electric blankets, computers, heated waterbeds, microwave ovens, cellular phones, and the like. For years scientists assumed EMFs were harmless. However, in 1989, as a result of a number of studies, the Congressional Office of Technology Assessment concluded that it could not be assumed there are no risks from EMFs. Of the studies done so far, any findings that EMFs cause cancer have been inconsistent. So, the final word is not yet in. While we wait for that final word, I will offer you the same precautions, from researchers at Carnegie-Mellon University, that I offered readers of my book *The Complete Book of Home Environmental Hazards,* published in 1990.

✿ ***What to do.***   Try to keep some distance from electrical appliances that are on all the time, such as an electric clock radio. Move it as far from your bed as possible. If you have an electric blanket, use it to warm the bed and turn it off before you get in. These are simple things you can do, with little, if any, inconvenience, until more information is in. Stay tuned (but, while you do, don't sit too near your radio or TV . . .). (See "Electromagnetic Field" in "Your Environment.")

✂ *Pesticides in Your Home*

Webster's defines pesticide as "any chemical used for killing insects, weeds, etc." The key word here is killing. If pesticides are poisonous to insects, which are much smaller than we are, could they be harmful to us as well? Could they kill us?

Pesticides are used in approximately 70 million homes in the United States. Eighty-five percent of the 84.5 million households average three to four pesticide products. There are over 20,000 different household pesticide products, containing over 300 active ingredients and as many as 1,700 inert ingredients, according to the National Home and Garden Pesticide Use Survey, done in 1990 for the Environmental Protection Agency (EPA) by the Research Triangle Institute. In 1993, 140,000 pesticide exposures, 93 percent of which involved home use, were reported to poison-control centers. EPA health statistician Jerome Blondell says that statistic may be the tip of the iceberg and that we could be misdiagnosing or overlooking the chronic effects caused by some of today's common household pesticide products.

Many of the pesticides in use today were developed after World War II, when a lot of new chemicals became available and were put on the market. At first pesticides were looked upon as miraculous. Suddenly you were able to get rid of bugs like termites, which could eat you out of house and home, and pesticide use on farms resulted in instantly higher yields of crops.

Pesticides have been regulated since the late 1940s. In 1947 the Federal Insecticide, Fungicide, and Rodenticide Act (FIFRA) was passed, providing regulation for the registration or licensing of pesticide products. The Environmental Protection Agency is now responsible for seeing that FIFRA is carried out. All pesticides sold in the United States must be approved by the EPA.

One potent pesticide, DDT, was banned in 1971, when it was found that it could remain in the environment indefinitely and move up the food chain from plant to animal and eventually to us. The possible role of DDT in the development of breast cancer is currently being investigated.

Disinfectants used to kill bacteria, fungi, and viruses account for the largest pesticide use in homes. Many people routinely use disinfectants, not to destroy bacteria or germs, but simply to clean. Formaldehyde is used in many commercial products for its disinfectant properties. In early 1992 formaldehyde was classified as a possible human carcinogen.

ℰ✎ *What to do.* For cleaning, always use a product that is nontoxic (check the label) unless there is a specific reason why a disinfectant is needed. Limit pesticide use in your home to as great an extent as possible.

NONTOXIC WAYS TO ELIMINATE BUGS AND PLANT DISEASE

- Pests need water to survive, so get rid of their sources of water. Fix any plumbing that leaks, and do not let water sit anywhere in your home—for example, don't regularly leave dishes in the sink to soak or plants sitting in wet trays.
- Pests also need food for good health and overall survival. Make sure none is available to them. Store food in sealed glass or plastic containers. If you have a pet,

don't leave its food out for an extended period of time. Put garbage, especially food scraps, in a tightly covered, heavy-gauge garbage can.

- Use bug traps or biological controls that expose pests to natural enemies or disease microorganisms.
- Make a pest homeless. Caulk those cracks and crevices that only the smallest and most annoying critters can get through. Remove piles of wood from under or around your home.
- Make sure all the screening on your windows is intact and hole free.
- To keep your houseplants healthy, use mulch to stifle weed growth and maintain even soil temperature and moisture.
- Get plants that are resistant to disease. Check for those varieties in a gardening book or consult your local nursery.

If you must use a pesticide, do so with great care. Choose the one that is the least toxic. Read the directions and precautions carefully, and adhere to them. Do not buy any pesticide in large quantities. Get just the amount you'll be using right away. When using the pesticide, wear protective clothing and avoid using aerosol sprays and foggers, which can stay in the air. If you treat a room, leave the area for as long as recommended on the label or by the applicator, if a professional does it. When you do return, open the windows and thoroughly air out the room. When you have finished using the pesticide, follow the instructions on the label for safe disposal of the container.

If you are having a professional do the exterminating, make certain they are licensed. Ask them what exactly they'll be using and if it is possible to use something non-chemical for control. Choose the least toxic method.

What do they say about an ounce of prevention . . . ? It could be years before we know the real danger that various pesticides pose. Wouldn't it be nice to be able to look back and say, "Oh, no problem. I stopped using that ages ago"?

৪৯ *Radon*

You can't smell it, see it, or feel it. But it could kill you. Radon is a naturally occurring, invisible radioactive gas. It comes from uranium that exists naturally in the earth's soil and rocks. It can also come from industrial wastes, such as by-products of uranium or phosphate mining. When it is outside your home, it is virtually harmless. It dissipates into the air. It's a different story when radon is inside your home. When it enters, it becomes trapped and accumulates, sometimes reaching dangerous concentrations. The Environmental Protection Agency (EPA) estimates that radon may be responsible for 20,000 lung cancer deaths a year in the United States. The National Cancer Institute's estimate is lower, at 14,400 deaths. That is 10 percent of lung cancer deaths. Radon may also be the cause of up to 30 percent of the lung cancer cases in nonsmokers.

There has been concern over radon since the 1960s, when some homes in the West, built with material contaminated by waste from uranium mines, were found to have high levels of radon. Concern skyrocketed when it was discovered that radon could get into a home and be trapped there, endangering the people living there. This was discovered serendipitously in December 1984, when Stanley Watras, an engineer working on the construction of the Limerick Nuclear Plant in Pennsylvania, went to the company Christmas party. When he *entered* the plant, he set off alarms that had been installed to detect radioactive contamination on any worker *leaving* the plant. He was bringing radiation in! The source of the radiation turned out to be Watras's home. When his house was tested for radiation, his living room had the highest level of radon ever found in the United States—a level that put him at a 100 percent risk of getting lung cancer. The discovery made headlines and created panic.

Radon can enter your home in a number of ways, through dirt floors, cracks in concrete floors and walls, floor drains, sumps, and joints and tiny cracks or pores in hollow block walls. It can also get into your home through your water supply, although radon in the water is considered much less of a threat. Since natural radon comes from soil and rock, the location of your house will have an impact on the radon level. However, if your neighbor has tested for radon and has safe levels, it doesn't mean you will. You may think that if you live in a new house, you are better off. That is not necessarily the case. If your house is airtight for energy efficiency, as so many newer houses are, it's at a greater risk of having a high level of radon, because once any amount of the gas gets into the house, it has no way to leave. If your house is old with windows that let in drafts, radon that does get in can also get out, making it very unlikely that you will have a problem with radon. The way your house was built can also be a factor in how much radon can enter. For example, since radon comes from the ground, if your home is built without a basement or crawl space, on a flat slab of concrete (which can contain minute cracks), more radon may enter your living area, resulting in greater exposure for the inhabitants.

It is very important to check your home for radon. There are many easy and inexpensive home radon tests available that you can use. There are also tests that require a professional. Some states and localities provide detectors free of charge or at a nominal cost.

RADON TESTS

- *Charcoal Canister*—This is widely available commercially in home centers and hardware stores. It can also be ordered through the mail. It requires no special skills and is relatively inexpensive. You may have to use more than one to measure levels in different parts of the house. You put the canister in the house for three to seven days and then send it out for processing and evaluation.
- *Alpha-Track Detector*—This is widely available commercially in home centers and hardware stores. It can also be ordered through the mail. It requires no special skills and is relatively inexpensive. You keep it in your house for a minimum of two to four weeks or as long as a year, then send it out for processing and evaluation.
- *Grab Sampling*—This must be done by a professional and can cost several hundreds of dollars. Results are obtained quickly.
- *Continuous Radon Monitoring/Continuous Working Level Monitoring*—Both methods involve the use of an electronic detector to gather and store information in order to get an average radon reading over a period of

time. This monitoring must be conducted by a professional and requires special equipment. It can cost several hundred dollars.

- *Radon Progeny Integrating Sampling Unit*—This uses an air pump that pulls air through the sampler constantly. The unit is installed by a professional and remains on for three days or longer. At the end of the test, the operator removes the unit and brings it to a lab for analysis and evaluation.
- *Liquid Scintillation Spectrometer*—A professional uses this to measure radon in the water.

Again, the tests you can do yourself are the charcoal canister and the alpha-track detector. What you want to do first is use a short-term test to find out the probability of a radon problem. You should conduct the test in the lowest "livable" area in the house—the basement, if you have one—because that is where the level will be highest. Close all windows and doors twelve hours before the start of the test, and keep them closed as much as possible for the test's duration. If you are using more than one detector, be sure to write the location, time you started the test, and an identifying number on each device. Hopefully, you will find that the radon level in your house falls well within EPA guidelines, in which case you can forget you ever heard of radon.

EPA GUIDELINES FOR HOME AND RADON LEVELS

- greater than 1 WL (working level) or 200 pCi/l (picocuries per liter): Perform follow-up measurements as soon as possible and consider taking immediate action to reduce the level.

- 0.1–1 WL or 20–200 pCi/l: Perform follow-up measurements for three months or less.
- 0.02–0.1 WL or 4–20 pCi/l: Perform follow-up measurements for either one continuous year or no more than one week's duration during each of the next four seasons.
- less than .02 WL or 4 pCi/l: Follow-up measurement probably not necessary.

The EPA recommends taking action if the average of one long-term test or two short-term tests done in the lowest level of your home show levels of 4 pCi/l or 0.02 WL. If you measure hazardous radon levels, you must first find out how the gas is entering your home. The first thing you'll want to do is make a visual inspection to locate any places where the radon may be getting in. Since radon cannot be seen or smelled and can come in through cracks that may be too small to see, you may have to call in an expert for an assessment on how the radon is getting inside and what to do to keep it out.

There are various ways to reduce the radon in your home. They vary in complexity and cost. Some methods are designed to prevent radon from entering, while others are designed to get it out. In most cases a skilled professional can determine the best method and how to implement it. The method used should be designed specifically for your house. It's not unusual for a combination of methods to be used.

RADON REDUCTION METHODS

- *Natural Ventilation*—This is definitely first choice. You don't need an expert for this. All you have to do is open your windows. The area most in need of ventilation is the lowest level of your house, where the radon generally enters. This method does have some marked disadvantages. Your heating bill could double or triple in the winter, and your summer air-conditioning bill could also go up substantially. Also, leaving your windows open could pose security problems. This is an excellent quick, but often temporary, solution for most homes.

- *Forced Ventilation*—This method operates on the same principles as natural ventilation but uses a fan, or fans, to draw in outside air, instead of relying on natural air movement. A fan can be installed to continuously blow fresh air into the house through the existing central forced-air heating system or through protected intakes in the sides of the house. A fan can be installed to blow outdoor air into a crawl space. You should *not* use the fan to draw air *out,* because you run the risk of decreasing the air pressure inside your home and, in doing so, drawing in *more* radon. Forced ventilation is relatively inexpensive to set up.

- *Heat Recovery Ventilation (HRV)*—This is a more sophisticated way of ventilating the house and replacing radon-laden air with outside air. The device used is called a heat-recovery ventilator or air-to-air exchanger. The air that is coming in is warmed by the air that it's replacing. Ducted units are designed, installed, and balanced by experienced contractors. The cost can run to several thousand dollars, including installation. Less complex and costly units can sometimes be installed by the homeowner. HRV is only cost-effective when there is a big difference between the temperature inside the house and outside.

- *Covering Exposed Earth*—Covering exposed earth in the basement, storage areas, drain areas, sumps, and crawl space will reduce the flow of radon into your home. If you are skilled, you can do it yourself. Otherwise, get a contractor to do it. It is difficult to tell ahead of time how effective this will be, since radon can seep through openings too small to see. If you have an earth floor in your basement, it should first be excavated, and before the concrete is poured, four inches of crushed stone should be put down. All joints must be carefully sealed. This should be checked regularly, since new openings can develop as the house settles.

- *Sealing Cracks and Openings*—This may do the trick for homes with marginal levels of radon. For sealing to be effective, it requires careful preparation of the area and controlled application of appropriate sealers. If you are not skilled, it's a good idea to have this done by a professional. Because it is usually not possible to find all the cracks and openings, the radon level may not be reduced as much as you had hoped it would be. In addition, new cracks and openings may occur. The EPA does not recommend the use of sealing alone to reduce radon, because, by itself, it has not been shown to lower radon levels significantly or consistently.

- *Drain-Tile Suction*—This method works best with houses whose foundations are encircled by drain tiles—perforated pipes that drain water away from the foundation, either to a drainage area or to a sealed sump. With the addition of a fan, these pipes can be used to pull radon from the surrounding soil and vent it away from the house. To add a fan to such a drainage system usually requires an experienced professional. This method will not be highly effective with houses that do not have complete drain-tile loops, or if some of the tiles are damaged or blocked. You or a professional should inspect any such system for these things before you rely upon it for radon removal.

- *Sub-Slab Suction*—This has been one of the most widely used and effective methods to pull radon from a house. Individual pipes are inserted under the foundation and a fan blows radon gas away from the foundation through the pipes. Houses with foundations that rest on aggregate soil (a cluster of very small soil granules) or highly permeable soil (soil that can be easily penetrated) are the best candidates for this method. The pipes can be inserted vertically or horizontally, and in most cases you should have an expert to install them.

- *Block-Wall Ventilation*—This method is only for homes that have walls made of hollow concrete blocks and is generally done by a professional. It can operate in one of two ways: wall suction can be employed, which draws radon from the spaces within the concrete block walls before it can enter the house, or wall pressurization, which blows air into the blocks, so that radon is prevented from entering the walls. This is a very effective method.

- *Prevention of House Depressurization*—The lower the air pressure in your house, compared to that in the soil, the more radon will be drawn in. Depressurization, a lowering of air pressure in the house, can be caused by an exhaust fan pushing inside air out or by a combustion unit, such as a fireplace or woodstove, that consumes air. There are some causes of depressurization that can be eliminated easily by the homeowner at very little cost. Your best bet on this one is to consult an expert.

- *House Pressurization*—In this method air pressure in the basement or crawl space is increased so that it is greater than that of the air in the soil under the house. The most common way of doing this is to blow air from upstairs into the basement or crawl space. This can only be done in houses that have a basement or heated crawl space that is tightly sealed from the living area. Installation requires an experienced contractor or a very skilled homeowner.

If you are not doing the radon reduction yourself, you will have to find a radon specialist to do the work. Many states now have lists of people qualified to do this. Some states have certification programs. If you want to hire a professional, call your state radon agency and ask for a list of certified or approved contractors and a copy of applicable state regulations.

ENGAGING A CONTRACTOR

- Obtain evidence of the contractor's experience and/or training in radon mitigation.
- Ask for and check out their references from previous clients.
- Get a written estimate. It's not a bad idea to get several estimates, as prices can vary, sometimes substantially.
- Get a second opinion from another contractor or a local government radiological health official if possible.
- Request specific details on what method will be used and why and how much the radon level will be reduced.

- Find out what the contractor will do if the levels are still too high after completion of the job.
- Inquire about what kind of guarantee is given for the work that is completed.

You also want to know the cost-effectiveness of the method being used. Sometimes another method that costs slightly more will give you a much greater reduction.

ৰ **What to do.**   Radon is a very dangerous, naturally occurring substance. If it's present in your home, it can pose a big threat. But if your home does have unacceptable levels of radon, there are many ways to reduce it. Doing so could save your life.

ৰ *Secondhand Smoke (environmental tobacco smoke)*

This is the smoke you are exposed to when you share your air with someone who is smoking. It is a combination of sidestream smoke (from the burning end of a cigarette as it smolders) and exhaled mainstream smoke (smoke that is breathed out by the smoker). In 1992 the U.S. Environmental Protection Agency (EPA) classified secondhand smoke as a Group A carcinogen, a category reserved for only the most dangerous cancer-causing agents. If you do not smoke and live with someone who does, your risk of developing lung cancer increases by about 30 percent. It is estimated that secondhand smoke is responsible each year for about three thousand lung cancer deaths in the United States. The more secondhand smoke you're exposed to, the greater your risk.

AVOIDING SECONDHAND SMOKE

In your home

- If any household member smokes, ask him or her not to smoke indoors. If your request is refused, ask the smoker to smoke in just one area of the house.
- Ask the smoker to smoke by an open window.
- Remove ashtrays to deter visitors from lighting up.
- Ask visitors not to smoke in your home.

In other places

- If you are at someone else's home, politely tell people there that you'd appreciate it if they would not smoke while you're there.
- If you are surrounded by smokers on the job, find out what local or state smoking regulations apply to the workplace and ask supervisors to enforce them.
- If smoking is permitted in your workplace, give your employer copies of reports on the harmful health effects of secondhand smoke.
- Ask to work near other nonsmokers and as far away from smokers as possible.
- Ask smokers, politely, if they would not smoke around you.
- Use a fan and open windows, when possible, to keep the air moving.

- Volunteer to help develop a fair company policy that protects nonsmokers.

&◆ **What to do.** This is something over which you do have some control. You may feel uncomfortable telling someone that smoking is not allowed in your home, but a diagnosis of lung cancer is far more uncomfortable! This is your call and your opportunity to take responsibility for your health.

|&◆ *Workplace Risks*

According to some epidemiological studies, the type of work a woman does may increase her risk of breast cancer. The Centers for Disease Control and Prevention reviewed some 2.9 million women's death certificates from 1979 through 1987. The study found that professional women, such as executives, teachers, librarians, and religious workers, had the highest incidence of breast cancer, while homemakers and women in military service, farming, and transportation had the lowest rate. Epidemiologist Carol Burnett says the most likely explanation is "delayed childbirth by professional women" and not toxic factors on the job. Dr. Paul Seligman, of the National Institute of Occupational Safety and Health, agrees, saying that the occupational risk has more to do with the delayed pregnancies of so many professional women. A study done in Vancouver, Canada, found that women who worked in data processing, food processing, insurance, and transportation had an elevated risk for breast cancer, although it did not conclude why this was seen.

Researchers at the University of North Carolina at Chapel Hill found that women in electrical occupations (electrical engineers, technicians, telephone installers, repairers, and line workers) had 38 percent excess mortality from breast cancer relative to other employees. The study, published in June 1994, was conducted to test the hypothesis that risk of breast cancer is increased by electromagnetic fields. The investigators acknowledged possible study limitations. Although they believed the findings were broadly consistent with other evidence supporting the association, they still urged further investigation.

You may increase your risk of developing cancer if you work at a beauty salon. Several studies of beauticians and other people who apply hair dye to others as part of their work have shown them to be at an increased risk of non-Hodgkin's lymphoma, multiple myeloma, and leukemia. The International Agency for Research on Cancer, a research organization that classifies exposures as carcinogenic to humans, has classified cosmetology as an occupation entailing exposures that are possibly carcinogenic.

𝕭 *What to do.* Depending on your particular concerns about conditions in your workplace, you have various options. Check on your state's smoking regulations for the workplace. Find out if the building has been tested for radon and asbestos. If you are in an occupation that appears to possibly have a higher rate of a particular cancer (bear in mind that there are virtually no definitive studies), you will have to weigh the possible risks against the known benefits of your situation.

III

Your Environment

It's been known for several centuries that cancer can be caused by exposure to elements that exist in the environment. In her book *Silent Spring*, which was published in 1962, biologist Rachel Carson wrote, "For the first time in the history of the world, every human being is now subjected to contact with dangerous chemicals, from the moment of conception until death." How many cancer deaths are actually caused by pollution in the environment? It's not known, and estimates made by scientists vary widely.

℘ *Air Pollution*

The source of most air pollution is modern industry and technology. Chemical plants, cars, manufacturing facilities, sewage treatment plants, and gas stations all contribute to this problem, spewing pollution into the air, including known carcinogens.

A major study done in 1985 by the Environmental Protection Agency (EPA) assessing the effects of air pollution, concluded that fifteen to forty-five air pollutants may be responsible for between 1,300 and 1,700 cancer cases a year in the United States. This is not a large number when compared to the total number of cancer cases a year, but you want to avoid being part of it.

According to a 1992 EPA air quality report, Spokane, Salt Lake City, Denver, Provo, and Chicago were the

U.S. cities whose air registered the highest levels of particulates, tiny bits of soot and ash from incinerators, factories, utility-company smokestacks, and diesel trucks. These particulates are possibly carcinogenic.

<u>WAYS TO PROTECT YOURSELF FROM BAD AIR</u>

- On smoggy days, restrict any strenuous outdoor activity to the early morning or early evening hours.
- Keep your car windows closed when driving in heavy traffic or through a tunnel.
- Take public transportation or carpool whenever possible.

&ə *What to do.*   Indoor air pollution, in your home or workplace, is a much greater health hazard than outdoor air pollution. However, you should take any steps possible to limit your exposure to outdoor air pollution. Check with your local health department on clean air regulations, and advise health officials if you believe they are not being adhered to. If you are shopping for a house, check with the local health department to see if there are toxic waste sites in the area. Check the street you'll be living on for the amount of its traffic spewing toxic fumes into the air.

&ə *Chemicals*

"Recent and unwelcome," is how David Ozonoff, M.D., at the Boston University School of Public Health, describes the chemicals in our environment. The chemical environment we live in today is a far cry from that of our grandparents. Before World War II our exposure to toxic chemicals was limited, because we didn't have the ability to make massive quantities of chemicals. Today, more than seventy thousand chemicals are being used in the United States.

In its National Toxicology Program, the United States government has identified some thirty known carcinogens, including:

- *4-aminobiphenyl*—Used in rubber and in the manufacture of dyes. It currently has no commercial use in the United States. It has been linked with bladder cancer.
- *analgesic mixtures containing phenacetin*—Used for over eighty years in drugs for mild to moderate pain in the muscles and bones. Phenacetin is not now being used in analgesics in the United States. Analgesics with phenacetin have been linked to several cancers, including renal, transitional cell, and bladder.
- *arsenic and certain arsenic compounds*—Used in pesticides, herbicides, the manufacture of glass and ceramics, and the smelting of metal ores. It may be found in food and drinking water. It is no longer manufactured in the United States, but it is still being imported. It's been associated with lung, skin, liver, and other cancers.
- *asbestos*—See "Asbestos."
- *azathioprine*—A synthetic chemical used in the treatment of some autoimmune diseases and patients with organ transplants. It has been linked with non-Hodgkin's lymphoma, skin cancer, and other tumors in various organs.
- *benzene*—An industrial chemical used in the manufac-

ture of plastics, paints, and adhesives, and as an additive in gasoline. You may be exposed to it as a result of exhaust from cars and buses. Cigarette smoking may also be a significant source of benzene. The Consumer Product Safety Commission requires labeling on products containing more than 5 percent and on paint and thinning solvents containing 10 percent or more. Benzene has been associated with leukemia.

- *benzidine*—An industrial chemical used in the manufacture of dyes for sixty years. It is no longer made for sale in the United States. It has been linked with bladder cancer.
- *bis-chloromethyl ether and technical-grade chloromethyl methyl ether*—Industrial chemicals used in the manufacture of plastics. They are associated with lung cancer.
- *1,4-butanediol dimethanesulfonate (Myleran)*—A drug used to treat some forms of leukemia. Some studies have indicated it may lead to the development of leukemia.
- *chlorambucil (Leukeran)*—A drug used to treat some forms of leukemia, lymphomas, and other cancers. Some studies have indicated it may lead to the development of leukemia.
- *chromium and chromium compounds*—A metal used as a protective coating for cars and equipment, in the tanning and textile industries, and in paint, food, and industrial water treatment. Studies have shown exposure can result in an increased risk of lung and other cancers.
- *conjugated estrogens*—A mixture of naturally occurring forms of estrogen used in the treatment of a num-

ber of conditions, including breast and prostate cancer. (See "Hormone Replacement Therapy.")

- *cyclophosphamide (Cytoxan, CTX, endoxan, Neosar)*—An anticancer drug used in the treatment of malignant melanoma, myeloma, leukemia, lymphoma, neuroblastoma, Ewing's sarcoma, and mycosis fungoides. Studies have shown that treatment with this drug can increase the risk for bladder cancer, leukemia, and other cancers.
- *DES (diethylstilbestrol)*—See "DES."
- *melphalan (Alkeran, L-PAM, phenylalanine mustard, L-phenylalanine mustard, L-sarcolysin)*—An anticancer drug used in the treatment of breast and ovarian cancer and myeloma. People treated with it face an increased risk of developing second primary cancers, mainly leukemia.
- *methoxsalen with ultraviolet A (PUVA) therapy*—A naturally occurring substance produced by several plants and a fungus. It is used to treat the skin diseases vitiligo and psoriasis and the cancer mycosis fungoides. It increases the risk of squamous cell carcinoma ninefold.
- *mustard gas*—An odorless, colorless, oily liquid that was used in chemical warfare during World War I. Studies have shown increased mortality from respiratory tract cancer among people exposed to it.
- *2-naphthylamine*—An industrial chemical used in the past in the manufacture of dyes. It has been associated with bladder cancer.
- *vinyl chloride*—A substance used industrially because of its flame retardant properties, its wide variety of end-use products, and its cost effectiveness. There is no evidence that exposure to any level of vinyl chloride is safe. Studies have shown increased risk of various

cancers, including lung, liver, brain, and lymphoma among people working with it.

The list of suspected carcinogens is much longer. According to Joan D'Argo of Greenpeace, most of the tens of thousands of chemicals in use have not been effectively tested and regulated. Samuel Epstein, M.D., professor of occupational and environmental health at the University of Illinois at the Medical Center in Chicago, says we are being exposed to tremendous environmental hazards. He cites an extensive body of evidence, including

- Production and manufacture of synthetic organic chemicals, particularly industrial carcinogens, went from one billion pounds in 1940 to over 400 billion pounds annually by the 1980s.
- Just 10 percent of the new chemicals have been adequately tested for carcinogenicity.
- Of some 120 substances identified as carcinogens in experiments in animals over the last twenty years, less than 10 percent have been subjected to epidemiological study by the NCI or industry.

When the EPA gauges the safety of pesticides, it uses tests that assume different chemicals do not interact with each other or have an additive effect when two or more chemicals are used together.

One reason chemicals may be so hazardous to us, as women, is the ability of so many of these chemicals to mimic estrogen. A study published in the fall of 1993 looked at previous studies on the possible link between chemicals that can act like estrogen, such as DDT, and

other organochlorines and breast cancer. The authors of
the study called for the development of major epidemiological studies to evaluate whether the incidence of
breast cancer is increasing because of increased exposure
to these chemicals. Most of the breast cancer risk factors,
such as the early onset of menstruation, late age of menopause, late or no pregnancy, and caloric intake can be
associated with a woman's total exposure to estrogen over
a lifetime. If exposure to chemicals can increase the total
amount of exposure to estrogen a woman faces, decreasing that exposure, as was done in Israel, may serve as a
way to reduce risk and prevent some breast cancers. In
the mid-1970s, consumers in Israel put pressure on the
Israeli government to take action against pesticides. The
government complied, phasing out the use of organochlorine pesticides at dairy farms. One study found that
breast cancer mortality rates dropped overall 8 percent
between 1976 and 1986. The authors of the study contend that the true rate of decrease was probably nearly
20 percent, if trends seen before the ban were factored
in.

On Long Island, where the breast cancer rate is significantly higher than the national rate, a study by the
New York State Department of Health reported in 1994
that women who once lived near large chemical plants
had a greater risk of developing breast cancer after menopause. Women who lived less than a mile from plants
producing chemical, rubber, and plastics between 1965
and 1975 had a greater than 62 percent increased risk of
getting breast cancer, with the risk increasing as the
number of neighboring chemical plants grew. Dr. Itzhak
Goldberg, chairman of the radiation oncology department at Long Island Jewish Medical Center, cited the

study as a "wake-up call for all of us." Goldberg said, "This study puts the issue on the front burner." Mary Wolff, Ph.D., associate professor of community medicine at Mt. Sinai School of Medicine in New York, called the study the "first credible report of its kind," a comment echoed by other researchers. She said that even though a link between the chemicals and the breast cancer was not established, the study nevertheless "casts suspicion in that direction, and that has to be followed up with more research." According to Mark Chassin, the New York State health commissioner, if the association between exposure to chemical production and the occurrence of breast cancer proves to be real, "it will be the first time that an environmental risk factor that is avoidable has been identified." Chassin also said that the findings could account for up to 5 percent of the breast cancer cases on Long Island. He qualified that by saying that he still believed the traditionally accepted risk factors, such as early menstruation, late birth of first child, late menopause, etc., could account for the higher rate of breast cancer there if a greater proportion of women living on Long Island had those risk factors than women in other locations. Previous studies on Long Island, including one by the CDC, had failed to find any environmental cause for the higher rate of breast cancer there.

In 1995 scientists from the NCI and the National Institute of Environmental Health Sciences (NIEHS) started a five-year intensive environmental study on Long Island. Created by congressional mandate in response to the loudly voiced concerns of Long Island residents about the high incidence of breast cancer there, the Long Island Breast Cancer Study Project (LIBCSP) calls for a study to assess "biological markers for environmental and other risk factors contributing to the incidence of breast cancer on Long Island." Schoharie County in New York and Tolland County in Connecticut, where breast cancer rates are elevated, are also part of the study. Iris Obrams, M.D., director of the study, says it presents "an opportunity for groundbreaking epidemiologic research that may serve, ultimately, as a research model for the nation." The study will look at past and current exposures of women (with and without breast cancer) to contaminated drinking water, indoor and ambient air pollution (including aircraft emissions and pesticide levels in the dust in household carpeting), electromagnetic fields, and hazardous and municipal wastes.

In April 1993 the NCI announced a number of ongoing or new studies looking at the possible link between breast cancer and environmental factors, including electromagnetic fields, pesticides, and contaminants in the food and water supply. In Michigan, where contamination of animal feed with PBBs (fat-soluble, cancer-causing substances formerly used as fire retardants) in the mid-1970s led to widespread contamination of farm animals, milk, and residents in the area, researchers will compare the levels of PBB residues in the breast fat of women with breast cancer with that of women without cancer.

From about 1947 to 1971, residents in a rural area of Alabama were exposed to high levels of DDT, when a chemical company discharged tons of the insecticide into a nearby river. People in the area regularly ate fish caught in the river. When the CDC investigated the population's blood levels of DDE (a by-product of DDT), they were about ten times higher than the average level found in people living in locations elsewhere in the country. The NCI is planning a case-control study to compare DDE residues in breast fat and blood of women with and without breast cancer.

🍞 ***What to do.*** There isn't much you can do other than educate yourself on what is in your neighborhood, such as a toxic waste site or a manufacturer who may be emitting hazardous chemicals into the water supply or air. If you are concerned about any of your findings, check with your local EPA office or department of health to find out what the current emissions regulations are and if they are being adhered to.

🍞 *Electromagnetic Field (EMF)*

EMFs are a combination of electric fields and magnetic fields that radiate from electrical cables, power lines, wires, fixtures, and appliances. Although studies continue on the possible role that EMFs emitted by electric power lines may play in the development of cancer, there are few conclusions. A Swedish study published in 1993, in which about half a million participants were followed over a long period of time, reported a doubling of the childhood leukemia rate in children exposed to EMFs. In Sweden it is now proposed that a standard be set that would require a 400-kilovolt power line to have 150 feet on each side as a buffer zone within which people could not live and schools could not be located.

There are a number of EMF studies that are currently underway. The University of Washington is conducting a study on EMFs and breast cancer. Patricia Coogan,

M.P.H., at the Boston University School of Public Health, is looking at breast cancer risk in women exposed to EMFs at work. Coogan says that the association of EMF emissions and breast cancer is plausible, because it is hypothesized that EMFs disrupt the functioning of the pineal gland, which produces melatonin. Melatonin inhibits the synthesis of estrogen and prolactin in the body, so a lowered level of melatonin may mean an increased level of exposure to estrogen, which would put a woman at a greater risk of breast cancer.

However, in April 1995, the American Physical Society, the world's largest group of physicists, said it could find no evidence that EMFs from power lines cause cancer. The society called the public's fear groundless and criticized the fact that billions of dollars were being spent for mitigation work to alleviate or lessen the concern when "more serious environmental problems are neglected for lack of funding." It concluded that "the conjectures relating cancer to power line fields have not been scientifically substantiated."

What to do. Although there certainly is not enough evidence to warrant selling your home if you are close to power lines, if you are buying a home, you may not want to get one where there is a lot of exposure to electric power lines, just in case. (See "Electromagnetic Field" in "Your Home and Workplace.")

ℰ Hazardous Waste Sites

O ne hundred tons of hazardous waste is produced in the United States each day! While that is a small part of the 6 billion tons of garbage generated yearly, it is definitely the most significant part. Industrial chemical waste is the most common source of hazardous substances, posing a threat to the environment and to those of us exposed to it.

There have been numerous accounts of the devastating effects of hazardous waste sites. One of the most well known is Love Canal, in upstate New York. Twenty-two thousand tons of chemical wastes, including polychlorinated biphenyls (PCBs), dioxin, and various long-lasting pesticides were dumped in the area by the Hooker Chemical Company. In 1953 Hooker filled in the dump and sold it to the city of Niagara Falls for one dollar. A road and houses were built, as well as a public school. Parents complained of nauseating smells, black sludge, and minor burn marks on their children. There were reports of an above average number of cases of breast cancer, leukemia, miscarriages, and birth defects. The cries were ignored until the late 1970s, when New York State started an investigation. In 1980 President Jimmy Carter declared a health emergency when an Environmental Protection Agency (EPA) study showed that a third of the residents had suffered chromosome damage. In 1985, 1,300 former Love Canal residents divvied up the $20 million awarded in their class-action suit. But that money meant little to Marie Pozniak who has cancer and whose daughter was born with abnormalities. Pozniak says that "any amount of money won't compensate for the mental anguish I face every time I look at my daughter."

The impact of any hazardous waste site depends on a number of different factors, including the toxicity of the chemicals, their concentration, and their location. Groundwater is most frequently contaminated, followed by surface water and air. Many of the waste sites are in locations where they seep into underground water and nearby streams and lakes. At some sites, toxic vapors rise from evaporating liquid wastes and pollute the air. Or the air becomes contaminated from uncontrolled chemical reactions. More than 25,000 hazardous waste sites have been reported to the EPA.

A survey in the early 1970s of new cancers in nine regions of the country, conducted by the National Cancer Institute, led to publication of "cancer maps." These maps show that an excess of many cancers, affecting both men and women, are clustered in regions of heavy industrialization and petrochemical plants.

The federal government has taken a number of steps to regulate toxic wastes. In 1980 Congress passed the Comprehensive Environmental Response, Compensation, and Liability Act (CERCLA) to, among other things, develop priorities for cleaning up the worst sites. The Toxic Substances Control Act (TSCA) requires the identification and control by the EPA of chemical products that pose a risk to humans or the environment through their manufacture, distribution, use, or disposal. The Resource Conservation and Recovery Act (RCRA) was set up to create guidelines for the management of toxic waste and its disposal.

What to do. If you suspect that an area near you may be a hazardous waste site, call your local health department, EPA office, or the RCRA hot line at (800) 424–

9346 and report it. You can find out about contaminants that may be coming your way from a nearby manufacturing plant or business. Any facility manufacturing hazardous chemicals must file that information with the Occupational Safety and Health Administration (OSHA). In your home, you can test the water for contamination from a nearby toxic waste site. Check with your local health department. If they do not test the water, they can direct you to someone who does. It's also a good idea to check any nearby pond or stream, especially if you fish or swim there. If you are buying a house, check with the local health department to find out the location of any toxic waste sites and avoid those areas.

℘ Pesticides in the Environment

Pesticides are another source of potentially hazardous chemicals in our environment. Used in agriculture, they pollute the air and contaminate the food supply and groundwater. Farm and factory workers who are exposed to large amounts of pesticides may face an increased risk of cancer. The Agricultural Health Study in Iowa and North Carolina (both states have a large population of farmers using pesticides) will assess exposures to agents such as pesticides, chemical solvents, engine exhausts, animal viruses, and sunlight in one hundred thousand farmers, their spouses and children. As cancer cases are diagnosed, breast cancer cases will be incorporated into special studies to collect even more detailed information on possible exposures and risk factors.

🍃 ***What to do.*** If you live in an area where there is widespread use of pesticides, take the precautions listed earlier in "pesticides in foods" and/or call the EPA pesticide hot line at (800) 858–PEST.

🍃 Pesticides on Your Lawn or Garden

Homeowners in the United States use ten times more pesticides per acre on their lawns and gardens than farmers do on their crops! According to a report from the National Academy of Sciences in 1990, homeowners use an estimated five to ten pounds of pesticides per acre of lawn each year or 300 million pounds. Of the most frequently used pesticides on lawns, twelve are suspected carcinogens. Even with the most careful use, some of the pesticides can drift into your home or onto the vegetables in your garden. And the pesticides can get into your water as well. In the EPA's National Pesticide Survey of private and public drinking-water wells, the chemical most often detected was a breakdown of the pesticide dacthal (DCPA), used primarily on lawns.

Some pesticides have the ability to stay in your body once they get in. They make themselves at home in your fat cells. In a woman's body, those pesticides can mimic estrogen and produce estrogenic effects. There is a lot of evidence that the greater the amount of contaminants contained in the fat in your body, the more harmful they are. The major contaminants of fat fall into these two categories: organochlorine pesticides, such as DDT (and its metabolite DDE), and other estrogenic pesticides, such as methoxychlor, toxaphene, dieldrin, endosulfan, chlordane, and aldrin. As many as thirty years ago some were shown to induce breast cancer in rodents. If the theory that as estrogen in the body increases, so does a woman's risk of breast cancer, is true, then exposure to pesticides (which end up as an estrogenlike compound in fatty breast tissue) may very well be a significant risk factor in the development of breast cancer.

A study in 1986 by the National Cancer Institute suggested that 2,4-D, a weed killer in common use, significantly increased the rate of non-Hodgkin's lymphoma in farmers who used it at least twenty days a year. We know from twenty studies in eight different countries that farmers and gardeners are at an increased risk of some cancers, which we think is related to their exposure to pesticides. Dogs whose owners use pesticides die at increased rates from certain cancers. However, a lush, green, and healthy "blue ribbon" lawn can be yours without the harmful effects of pesticides, with a minimal effort on your part.

<u>GARDEN AND LAWN CARE WITHOUT PESTICIDES</u>

Make a needs assessment

- Evaluate your lawn and garden for pests and injuries to plants, amount of sunlight and water available, adaptation of plants and trees to the site.

Soil care

- Test annually for fertility and pH level; fertilize twice in the fall and once in the spring.
- If soil gets less than one inch of rainfall per week, water once each week; water deep, to encourage extensive root growth.
- Use a "soil activator" once or twice a year to enrich and stimulate the microbial life in the soil.
- Use compost. As it breaks down, it releases vital nutrients into the soil. You can buy it in garden stores or from a local farmer, or make it yourself from old bread, coffee grounds, vegetables, peels, egg shells, and used paper products. It is easy to make a compost bin in your backyard with some scrap wood, chicken wire, snow fencing, or cinder block.

Physical care

- Your mower should be set to mow grass to a height of between three and four inches. A lawn at that height may limit the growth of weeds, especially crabgrass, and is less susceptible to insect pests and disease.
- Prune trees and shrubs regularly, removing plant parts that are pest or disease infested.
- Regularly remove weeds and their roots to extend the range of healthy grass.
- Spray your lawn weekly with a water hose to dislodge aphids and other common garden pests.
- Use mulch to create physical barriers for weed control around garden plants.

Insects, birds, and other biological controls

- Assess which of the insects are actually the good guys and which are the pests. In a residential setting, insects such as ladybugs, lacewings, bees, dragonflies, praying mantises, and nematodes feed on the insects considered to be pests. For example, you won't want to rid your lawn and garden of the spined soldier bug, which can feed on more than one hundred insect pests.
- Bacillus thuringiensis (Bt) is a naturally occurring bacteria that acts as a form of biological control. It is available in a dust or spray under various commercial trade names. It is frequently applied to trees and vegetation to control caterpillars in parks and other recreation areas.
- Birds will flock to certain trees, shrubs, and plants and act as a natural regulator of insects. Find out about the local bird population and how to attract the good birds to your property.

Planning planting

- Grasses and plants most likely to be resistant to pests and disease are those that are native to the region.

✍ **What to do.**   Go the natural way and avoid pesticide use to as great an extent as possible. Just as there are bad pests that can wreak havoc in your yard, there are good guys that can help you get rid of those bad guys. Your county agricultural extension service can be an excellent source of helpful information on which is which.

| &ə *Radiation*

I t's been known for decades that radiation can cause cancer. It wasn't understood that very small amounts of radiation, such as fallout from bomb testing in the 1950s and 1960s and small releases from nuclear reactors (military and commercial), had harmful effects. However, large increases in cancer rates in different countries and different parts of the country appear to have occurred since such testing began. Epidemiological studies show a relationship with cancer occurrence when emissions from nuclear reactors in different regions are compared with incidence of cancer in those regions.

In Japan, five to seven years after the bombing of Hiroshima and Nagasaki, a twenty- to twenty-fivefold increase was seen in such leukemias as acute lymphocytic (ALL), acute myelogenous (AML), and chronic myelogenous (CML) among atomic bomb survivors. A study of people exposed to radioactive fallout from nuclear tests in Nevada during the 1950s showed a slight increase in the incidence of acute leukemias in people under twenty over that in the general population. Patients who received at least two grays (a measurement used for the amount of radiation absorbed by the body) of radiation as a treatment for ankylosing spondylitis (a painful condition of the spine) have an increased incidence of AML. Individuals exposed to radiation or X-rays before birth have an increased risk of developing ALL by the age of fifteen.

Some data suggest that 5 to 10 percent of the patients treated with chemotherapy and radiation for Hodgkin's disease develop acute leukemia within two to twelve years after their first treatment.

୫ **What to do.** Make every effort to limit, to as great an extent as possible, your exposure to any radiation. If you are getting radiation treatment for cancer, its benefits, in general, outweigh any risks. But be sure to question the doctor about the equipment being used, the amount of radiation you'll be getting, and the possible side effects. Make sure the radiologic equipment at the facility is up to date. Ask your doctor the potential cancer risks of the radiation, so that you'll be aware and on the lookout for any possible signs of cancer. Again, with radiation treatment, the benefits usually greatly outweigh any risks.

୫ *Sunshine*

When I was growing up, sunshine was considered to be healthy. I can well remember the long, hot days at Jones Beach on Long Island, where my family would go every summer. I also remember the sunburns I suffered, some of them severe. Now I see a dermatologist every six months to be checked for new skin cancers. If I'd known then what we know today, I could have prevented my skin cancer. Because of what we now know, this is one risk factor that can be easily avoided, but *must be avoided early on,* because 80 percent of the skin damage that results in skin cancer occurs before the age of eighteen, and it cannot be undone. Sun-induced skin damage is cumulative and irreversible.

You are at the greatest risk for skin cancer if you are fair skinned, have red or blond hair, freckle easily, have blue or light-colored eyes, live in southern areas that get high levels of UV radiation from the sun, and have a long history of exposure to the sun. Nevertheless, there are things you can do to avoid increasing your risk of skin cancer. Of course, if you have children, it is extremely important that they be protected from exposure to the harmful rays. These tips are for everyone:

- Avoid exposure to the midday sun, 10 A.M. to 2 P.M. standard time or 11 A.M. to 3 P.M. daylight saving time.
- Use protective clothing, such as a sun hat with a brim and shirts with long sleeves.
- Use lotions that contain sunscreens to protect the skin. Sunscreens with a sun protection factor (SPF) of 15 to 30 block most of the sun's harmful rays.
- Avoid the use of tanning devices.

There is hope on the horizon for those who didn't take precautions. Researchers at Applied Genetics, in Freeport, New York, are working on a cream containing an enzyme to repair DNA damage within cells of the skin in order to prevent skin cancer. The cream is being tested on people with a rare, inherited condition called xeroderma pigmentosum. Their skin lacks the ability to repair damaged DNA, and about half of them develop skin cancer by the age of eight. If it works, it could eventually be available to the general public.

ɮ *What to do.* As with all cancer, the earlier skin cancer is detected the better the chance for a cure. If you think you may be a candidate for skin cancer, follow the advice of the American Cancer Society, which recommends skin self-examination by adults on a monthly basis. An annual examination by a physician is also rec-

Every Woman's Handbook for Preventing Cancer

ommended. Any signs or symptoms of skin cancer should be checked out. Once you are diagnosed with skin cancer, you are at an increased risk of developing subsequent skin cancers and should see a doctor regularly, every four to six months.

The Most Common Cancers Affecting Women in 1996

BLADDER CANCER

INCIDENCE: 14,600 per year
DEATHS: 3,900 per year
RISK FACTORS:
- smoking
- employment in the rubber, chemical, or leather industries, or as a hairdresser, machinist, metal worker, printer, painter, textile worker, or truck driver
- bladder infection caused by the parasitic flatworm Schistosoma haematobium
- long-term use of painkillers containing phenacetin (which is now banned by the FDA)
- drinking chlorinated water for over 40 years ✳

SYMPTOMS:
- blood in the urine, usually associated with increased frequency of urination (most common symptom)
- painful urination
- feeling or urgency to urinate
- retention of urine (rare)
- incontinence (rare)

SCREENING/DIAGNOSTIC TESTS: vaginal or rectal exam, urinalysis, CT scan, flow cytometry, cyctoscopy, biopsy

BREAST CANCER

INCIDENCE: 184,300 per year

DEATHS: 44,300 per year

RISK FACTORS:

- being age 40 or older, risk increases with age
- family history of cancer
- personal history of breast cancer
- personal history of ovarian cancer
- atypical hyperplasia
- early menstruation (before age 12)
- completion of menopause after age 55
- having first child when over the age of 30
- having no children
- obesity
- alcohol use
- a high-fat diet
- smoking
- hormone-replacement therapy (not well established)
- oral contraceptives taken at an early age

SYMPTOMS:

- a lump or thickening in or near the breast or in the under-arm area
- a change in the size or shape of the breast
- a discharge from the nipple
- a change in the color or feel of the skin of the breast, areola, or nipple (dimpled, puckered, or scaly).

SCREENING/DIAGNOSTIC TESTS: breast self-exam, clinical breast exam, mammography, ultrasound, biopsy

CERVICAL CANCER

INCIDENCE: 15,700 per year

DEATHS: 4,900 per year

RISK FACTORS:
- being age 18 or older
- sexual intercourse before age 18
- many sexual partners
- human papillomavirus (HPV), genital warts
- having a mother who took DES
- HIV infection
- oral contraceptives
- squamous intraepithelial lesion (SIL)
- cervical dysplasia
- first pregnancy before the age of 18 or multiple pregnancies

SYMPTOMS:
- abnormal uterine bleeding
- abnormal vaginal discharge

SCREENING/DIAGNOSTIC TESTS: Pap test, pelvic exam, colposcopy, biopsy

COLORECTAL CANCER

INCIDENCE: 65,900 per year
DEATHS: 27,500 per year
RISK FACTORS:
- being age 50 or over, risk increases with age
- low intake of foods containing fiber and high intake of fat
- consumption of mutagens produced when food, especially meat, is cooked at high temperatures
- family history of colorectal cancer
- excessive alcohol use
- familial adenomatous polyposis (FAP), Gardner's syndrome, Turcot's syndrome, or Oldfield's syndrome
- intestinal polyps
- severe obesity: 40 percent or more over your ideal weight

- hereditary nonpolyposis colorectal cancer (HNPCC) (Lynch syndromes I and II)

SYMPTOMS:
- diarrhea or constipation
- blood in or on the stool (either bright red or very dark)
- stools that are narrower than usual
- general stomach discomfort (bloating, fullness, cramps)
- frequent gas pains
- a feeling that the bowel doesn't empty completely
- loss of weight for no apparent reason
- constant tiredness
- unusual paleness

SCREENING/DIAGNOSTIC TESTS: digital rectal exam, sigmoidoscopy, occult blood stool test, colonoscopy, lower GI series, biopsy

KIDNEY CANCER

INCIDENCE: 12,100 per year
DEATHS: 4,700 per year
RISK FACTORS:
- smoking
- heavy, long-term use of the painkiller phenacetin (no longer sold in the United States)
- obesity
- working near a coke oven (an oven in which coke, an industrial fuel, is made)
- working with asbestos

SYMPTOMS:
- pain on one side of the back
- blood in the urine
- a mass in the abdomen
- high blood pressure
- fever

- loss of appetite (less common)
- nausea and vomiting (less common)
- constipation (less common)
- weakness (less common)
- fatigue (less common)

SCREENING/DIAGNOSTIC TESTS: intravenous pyelogram (IVP), CT scan, ultrasound, arteriogram, MRI, nephrotomography, biopsy

LEUKEMIA

INCIDENCE: 12,300 per year
DEATHS: 9,400 per year
RISK FACTORS:
- exposure to radiation
- radiation and chemotherapy used in the treatment of Hodgkin's disease
- exposure to electromagnetic fields
- a family history of leukemia
- having the Philadelphia chromosome (Ph[1])
- exposure to benzene (present in gasoline)
- the drugs chloramphenicol and phenylbutazone
- treatment with alkylating agents (a chemotherapy drug that interferes with the division process of cancer cells, slowing or stopping their growth and reproduction)

SYMPTOMS:
- fever and flulike symptoms
- enlarged lymph nodes
- enlarged spleen
- enlarged liver
- bone pain
- joint pain
- paleness
- weakness

- tendency to bleed or bruise easily
- frequent infections

SCREENING/DIAGNOSTIC TESTS: blood tests, bone marrow biopsy, spinal test, biopsy

LUNG CANCER

INCIDENCE: 78,100 per year
DEATHS: 64,300 per year
RISK FACTORS:
- smoking, smoking, smoking!
- exposure to secondhand smoke
- radon
- asbestos
- exposure in the workplace to bis-chloromethyl ether and chloromethyl methyl ether, chromium compounds, beryllium, arsenic
- chronic obstructive pulmonary disease (COPD)
- a defective p53 gene
- inheritance of a strong ability to metabolize the chemical debrisoquine (found in cigarette smoke)

SYMPTOMS:
- persistent cough, "smoker's cough"
- hoarseness
- difficulty swallowing
- increased sputum
- sputum streaked with blood
- coughing up blood
- constant chest pain
- labored breathing, shortness of breath
- recurring pneumonia or bronchitis
- swelling of the neck and face
- pain or weakness in the shoulder, arm, or hand

- fatigue
- loss of appetite
- weight loss

SCREENING/DIAGNOSTIC TESTS: chest X-ray, sputum cytology, bronchoscopy, biopsy, mediastinoscopy, thoracotomy

MELANOMA

INCIDENCE: 16,500 per year
DEATHS: 2,700 per year
RISK FACTORS:
- exposure to the sun, sunlamps, tanning booths
- having a fair complexion that freckles easily, blond or red hair, blue or light-colored eyes
- living in the South, where the sun is strongest
- having one or more blistering sunburns as a child or teenager
- dysplastic nevus syndrome
- two or more close relatives with melanoma
- familial atypical multiple mole melanoma (FAMMM) syndrome
- a high-fat diet

SYMPTOMS:
- a change in the size, shape, or color of a mole
- oozing or bleeding from a mole
- a mole that feels itchy, hard, lumpy, swollen, or tender to the touch

SCREENING/DIAGNOSTIC TESTS: Screening is done by a thorough examination of the body for any suspicious growths on the skin; diagnosis is by removing the growth and performing a biopsy

NON-HODGKIN'S LYMPHOMA

INCIDENCE: 22,800 per year
DEATHS: 10,900 per year

SYMPTOMS:
- painless swelling of the lymph nodes in the neck, groin, or underarm
- fevers
- night sweats
- tiredness
- weight loss
- itching
- reddened patches on the skin
- nausea (less common)
- vomiting (less common)
- abdominal pain (less common)

SCREENING/DIAGNOSTIC TESTS: thorough physical exam, complete blood test, X-rays, tomography, CT scan, urinalysis, bone marrow test, lymphangiography, biopsy

OVARIAN CANCER

INCIDENCE: 26,700 per year
DEATHS: 14,800 per year
RISK FACTORS:
- a family history of ovarian cancer
- being over 50 years of age
- having a history of breast cancer
- early menstruation (before age 12)
- completion of menopause after age 55
- never having children
- having first child after age 30
- severe obesity: 40 percent or more over your ideal weight
- diabetes

- high blood pressure
- Lynch syndrome II
- using the fertility drugs Clomid and Serophene and not getting pregnant

SYMPTOMS: Usually none in the early stages; varied symptoms may appear as the tumor grows.
- a swollen or bloated feeling, or general discomfort in the abdomen
- loss of appetite
- feeling of fullness, even after a light meal
- gas, indigestion, nausea
- weight loss
- diarrhea, constipation, or frequent urination
- shortness of breath

SCREENING/DIAGNOSTIC TESTS: pelvic examination, ultrasound, transvaginal ultrasonography, CA-125 test, biopsy

PANCREATIC CANCER

INCIDENCE: 13,900 per year
DEATHS: 14,200 per year
RISK FACTORS:
- smoking
- hereditary pancreatitis (inflammation of the pancreas)
- Gardner's syndrome
- a high-fat diet

SYMPTOMS: Early symptoms resemble those of other digestive disorders.
- nausea
- abdominal pain and discomfort
- belching
- a feeling of fullness
- intolerance for fatty foods

- weight loss
- loss of appetite
- loss of strength and energy

SCREENING/DIAGNOSTIC TESTS: ultrasound, CT scans, X-rays, endoscopic retrograde cholangiopancreatography, CA-19a, CEA assay, biopsy

SKIN CANCER—NONMELANOMA

INCIDENCE (men and women): over 800,000 basal and squamous cell per year
DEATHS (men and women): 2,100 deaths per year
RISK FACTORS:
- exposure to the sun, sunlamps, tanning booths
- having a fair complexion that freckles easily, blond or red hair, blue or light-colored eyes
- living in the South, where the sun is strongest
- having one or more blistering sunburns as a child or teenager
- a high-fat diet

SYMPTOMS:
- a change on the skin, especially a new growth or a sore that does not heal. (Although they can develop anywhere, squamous and basal cell skin cancers usually are found on areas of the skin that have been exposed to the sun.)

SCREENING/DIAGNOSTIC TESTS: Screening is done by a thorough examination of the body for any suspicious growths on the skin; diagnosis is by removing the growth and performing a biopsy

STOMACH CANCER

INCIDENCE: 8,800 per year
DEATHS: 5,700 per year
RISK FACTORS:
- being age 55 or older
- smoking
- Helicobacter pylori (a type of bacteria)
- pernicious anemia
- achlorhydria
- gastric atrophy
- consumption of foods containing nitrates, nitrites, and nitro-samines

SYMPTOMS:
- indigestion or a burning sensation (heartburn)
- discomfort or pain in the abdomen
- nausea and vomiting
- diarrhea or constipation
- bloating of the stomach after meals
- loss of appetite
- weakness and fatigue
- bleeding (vomiting blood or having blood in the stool)

SCREENING/DIAGNOSTIC TESTS: occult blood stool test, upper GI series, endoscopy, biopsy

UTERINE CANCER (ENDOMETRIAL CANCER)

INCIDENCE: 34,000 per year
DEATHS: 6,000 per year
RISK FACTORS:
- being age 55 to 70, risk increases with age
- early menstruation (before age 12)
- completion of menopause after age 55
- having few or no children
- diabetes

- obesity
- high blood pressure
- being of high socioeconomic status
- Lynch syndrome II
- atypical uterine hyperplasia

SYMPTOMS:

- staining or bleeding, especially after menopause

SCREENING/DIAGNOSTIC TESTS: pelvic exam, endometrial aspiration, Pap test, D & C, biopsy

Glossary

abdomen   The part of the body that contains the stomach, intestines, liver, reproductive organs, and other organs.

acceptable air quality   Air in which there are no known contaminants at harmful concentrations.

achlorhydria   A lack of hydrochloric acid in the digestive juices in the stomach, which can increase the risk for stomach cancer. Hydrochloric acid helps digest food.

adenoma   A benign tumor that grows on the surface of an organ or gland.

alkylating agents   Chemotherapy (anticancer drugs) that can interfere with the division process of cancer cells, stopping or slowing their growth and reproduction.

alpha-track detector   A device used to test for radon levels; it is a small container with a sheet of special plastic on which the concentration of radon can be registered and evaluated.

antioxidants   These are substances that slow or prevent the possible harmful effects of oxidation on foods and on cells in the body. Antioxidants may prevent the formation of free radicals, which have been linked to cancer.

arteriogram   An X-ray of blood vessels, which can be seen after injection of a dye; used most frequently in the evaluation of liver, pancreatic, or brain cancer.

asbestos A group of naturally occurring mineral fibers found in rocks and used in various building materials, including pipe and boiler insulation, woodstove gaskets, and some plaster products. When its fibers are inhaled, it can cause lung cancer, mesothelioma (cancer of the membrane lining the chest or lung), and other cancers.

barium enema Part of a lower GI (gastrointestinal) series exam, which is a series of X-rays of the lower intestine taken after the patient has been given an enema with a white, chalky solution that contains barium. A barium enema may be used in the diagnosis of colon cancer.

benign tumor An abnormal, noncancerous growth of tissue that does not spread to other parts of the body. A benign tumor may become cancerous.

biopsy Removal of a sample of tissue for microscopic examination for cancer cells.

bone marrow The soft, spongy tissue in the center of many bones. It produces white blood cells, red blood cells, and platelets.

bone marrow aspiration Removal of a sample of fluid and cells from the bone marrow by needle for microscopic examination for cancer cells. It may be used in the diagnosis of leukemia and other cancers.

bone marrow biopsy Removal of a sample of solid tissue from the bone marrow for microscopic examination for cancer cells. It may be used in the diagnosis of leukemia and other cancers.

bronchoscopy A procedure in which a lighted tube (bronchoscope) is inserted through the nose or mouth into the lungs so that the bronchi can be seen. It may be used in the diagnosis of lung and other cancers.

CA-125 A protein that can be measured in the blood. Elevated levels are found in 80 percent of women diagnosed with ovarian cancer. It can be used in the diagnosis of ovarian cancer and to monitor the effectiveness of treatment of ovarian cancer. An elevated level after treatment can indicate the recurrence of cancer. Testing for CA-125 may also be used with other gynecologic cancers but is most reliable for ovarian.

calcifications In breast tissue they are small calcium deposits that are found by mammography. Microcalcifications, which are tiny specks of calcium, may be an indication of breast cancer. Macrocalcifications, which are coarse calcium deposits, are associated with benign conditions most likely caused by aging or old injuries.

cancer A term for the more than one hundred diseases in which abnormal cells divide without control.

carcinoma in situ Cancer that involves only the cells in which it began and that has not spread to other tissues. In situ cancers are usually curable.

CAT scan (CT scan, computerized axial tomography) A series of detailed, cross-sectioned pictures of areas inside the body created by a computer linked to an X-ray machine. It may be used in the diagnosis of many cancers, including lung, brain, breast, bladder, uterine, ovarian, and pancreatic.

cauterization The use of heat to destroy abnormal cells. It may be used to treat abnormal cervical cells that may be precancerous.

CEA (carcinoembryonic antigen) assay A laboratory test used to measure the level of CEA, an antigen produced by some types of tumors. An increased amount in the blood may indicate the presence of colorectal or pancreatic cancer. The CEA may also be used to monitor some cancer patients. An elevated level could indicate that the treatment is not working or that the cancer has recurred.

cervical intraepithelial neoplasia (CIN) A term for the growth of abnormal cells on the surface of the cervix. Numbers from 1 to 3 are often used to describe how much of the cervix contains abnormal cells.

cervix The lower, narrow end of the uterus that forms a canal between the uterus and the vagina.

charcoal canister A device containing activated charcoal that absorbs radon gas. It is used to test for radon levels in a specific location in the home.

chemoprevention The use of specific anticancer drugs, chemicals, vitamins, or other natural or synthetic agents to reverse or suppress the development or progression of cancer (currently the NCI is sponsoring over thirty-five clinical trials on chemoprevention).

chemotherapy Treatment with anticancer drugs.

chronic obstructive pulmonary disease (COPD) A condition characterized by progressive limitation of the flow of oxygen into and out of the lungs. Emphysema and chronic bronchitis are forms of COPD. This is a risk factor for lung cancer.

clinical trial A study conducted with patients, usually to evaluate a new treatment. Each study is designed to answer scientific questions and to find better ways to treat patients or prevent disease.

colon The section of the large intestine above the rectum. The colon is also called the "large bowel" or "large intestine."

colonoscopy An examination in which the doctor looks at the colon through a flexible lighted instrument (colonoscope).

colorectal cancer (colon/rectal cancer) The presence of cancer cells in the colon, the rectum, or the cecum (the first part of the large intestine). Because the rectum is part of the colon, colon cancer and rectal cancer are often referred to as one.

colposcopy A procedure in which a lighted magnifying instrument (colposcope) is used to examine the vagina and cervix.

complete remission The disappearance of all signs and symptoms of cancer.

conization (cone biopsy) Removal of a cone-shaped piece of tissue, often from the cervix and cervical canal to diagnose or treat a cervical condition.

cryosurgery Treatment performed with an instrument that freezes and destroys abnormal tissue. It may be used in the treatment of liver, cervical, or skin cancer.

CT scan see "CAT scan."

cyst A sac or capsule in the body filled with fluid.

cystoscopy Insertion of a lighted instrument (cystoscope) into the urethra to look at the bladder.

D & C (dilation and curettage) A minor surgical procedure in which a small, spoon-shaped instrument (curette) is used to scrape the cervical canal and uterine lining. The cells that are removed can be biopsied and used in the diagnosis of cervical cancer.

DES (diethylstilbestrol) A drug, once widely prescribed to prevent miscarriages, that has been linked to cancer of the female reproductive system.

digital rectal exam A test in which the doctor inserts a lubricated, gloved finger into the rectum to feel for abnormal areas that can be a sign of rectal cancer.

dioxin A toxic by-product of chemical processes, such as the manufacture of pesticides or paper bleaching; it is also found in Agent Orange.

DNA (deoxyribonucleic acid) A nucleic acid that contains the genetic information of a cell, present in all living cells.

dysplasia Abnormal cells that are not cancerous but which may or may not become cancerous.

dysplastic nevi Moles whose appearance is different from that of common moles. In general they are larger, have irregular borders, color that is not uniform, and are flat. Dysplastic nevi are a risk factor for melanoma.

electromagnetic fields (EMFs) A combination of electric fields and magnetic fields that radiate from electrical cables, wires, fixtures, and appliances.

endometrium The layer of tissue that lines the uterus. Endometrial (uterine) cancer can develop there.

endoscope A flexible, lighted instrument used to examine organs or body cavities, such as the lungs, colon, cervix, bladder, small intestine, stomach, abdomen, throat, esophagus, and vagina.

endoscopic retrograde cholangiopancreatography (ERCP) A special X-ray of the common bile duct, which may be used in the diagnosis of pancreatic cancer.

endoscopy An examination using an endoscope.

erythroplakia (erythroplasia) A reddened patch with a velvety surface found in the mouth. It is considered a precancerous condition.

esophagus A muscular tube that carries food from the throat to the stomach.

estrogen The main female hormone.

fecal occult blood test see "occult blood stool test."

first-degree relative A mother, father, son, daughter, sister, or brother.

formaldehyde (HCHO) A colorless, gaseous compound with a detectable pungent smell at high concentrations. It can be used as a disinfectant or preservative. Exposure to formaldehyde may put a person at greater risk for some cancers, including nasopharyngeal, brain, lung, and leukemia.

free radicals Substances that are formed by oxidation in the body and can damage healthy cells, making them more vulnerable to cancer.

gastric atrophy A condition in which the stomach muscles shrink and become weak, leading to a lack of secretions needed for digestion. This may be a precursor of stomach cancer.

gastroscope A flexible, lighted instrument that is put through the mouth and esophagus to view the stomach. Tissue from the stomach for a biopsy can also be removed.

gene A biological unit composed of DNA; genes control all physical, biochemical, and physiologic traits.

genetic Inherited; having to do with information that is passed from parents to their children through DNA.

grab sampling A way of collecting an air sample to measure contaminant levels.

gynecologic oncologists Doctors who specialize in treating cancers of the female reproductive organs.

Helicobacter pylori Bacteria that cause inflammation and ulcers in the stomach. It is a risk factor for stomach cancer.

hormones Chemicals produced by the glands in the body. Hormones control the actions of certain cells or organs.

human papillomaviruses (HPV) Viruses that generally cause warts. Some HPVs are sexually transmitted and are thought to cause abnormal changes, which could become cancerous, in the cells of the cervix. Most women who are infected with HPV do not develop cervical cancer.

hyperplasia   A precancerous condition in which there is an abnormal increase in the number of normal cells in a tissue or organ.

hysterectomy   An operation in which the uterus and cervix are removed. A hysterectomy may be performed in the treatment of some cancers, including cervical, endometrial, and ovarian.

immune system   A network in the body that protects against disease-causing agents, such as bacteria, viruses, and cancer.

incidence   The number of new cases of a disease during a specific period.

indoor air pollution   The contamination by noxious gases or airborne particles, from any source, that makes indoor air unpleasant or unhealthy to breathe.

initiation   An event that causes a genetic mutation, predisposing a person to cancer.

intravenous pyelogram (IVP)   An X-ray study of the urinary tract, including the kidneys, ureters, and bladder.

invasive cancer (invasive carcinoma)   Cancer that has spread to healthy tissue adjacent to the tumor. It may or may not have spread to other parts of the body.

Krukenberg tumor   A tumor of the ovary caused by the spread of stomach cancer.

liquid scintillation spectrometer   A device for measuring radon levels in water.

lower GI series   see "barium enema."

lymphatic system   The tissues and organs that produce, carry, and store cells that fight infection. It includes the bone marrow, spleen, thymus, lymph vessels, and lymph nodes. Cancer that arises in the lymphatic system is known as lymphoma.

mainstream smoke   Smoke drawn through tobacco during inhalation and then exhaled.

malignant   Cancerous, capable of invading nearby tissues or spreading to other parts of the body.

mediastinoscopy   A procedure in which a tube (mediastinal scope) is inserted through an incision above the collarbone so that the organs of the mediastinum can be viewed. It is called a *mediastinotomy* when the incision is made on one side of the breastbone. It may be used in the diagnosis of lung cancer.

menopause   The time of a woman's life when menstrual periods permanently stop.

metastasis   The process by which malignant cells separate from the primary site and travel to another site in the body neither adjacent to nor connected to the original site.

monoclonal antibodies   Antibodies that are specific for a single antigen. They can be produced in large quantities in the laboratory and are being studied in clinical trials to determine their effectiveness in cancer detection, diagnosis, and treatment.

MRI (magnetic resonance imaging)   A procedure that uses a magnet linked to a computer to create pictures of areas inside the body. It is used in the diagnosis of many cancers.

neoplasia   Abnormal new growth of cells, which may be cancerous.

nephrectomy   Surgery to remove the kidney.

nephrotomogram   A series of special X-rays of the kidneys taken from different angles, which show the kidneys clearly, without the shadows of the organs around them.

nitrate A chemical substance used in the preservation of some foods that can change into nitrite and eventually nitrosamine, which is a carcinogen.

NK (natural killer) cells Large lymphocytes that attack certain cells on contact and probably help regulate the immune system.

occult blood stool test (fecal occult blood test) A simple, noninvasive screening test for blood in the stool, which may indicate the possibility of colorectal cancer. This test, though far from foolproof, can be an early warning sign and help in the detection of colorectal cancer when it is most curable. After you turn fifty, you should have this test every year.

oncogenic Capable of causing cancer.

oophorectomy The removal of one or both ovaries. Oophorectomy used to be performed in the treatment of breast cancer in premenopausal women. It has been replaced in most instances by hormonal therapy.

ovaries The pair of female reproductive organs that produce eggs and hormones. They are located in the lower abdomen, one on each side of the uterus.

palpation Feeling part of the body, for example the breast, with the fingers for signs of lumps or any other abnormalities that may indicate disease.

pancreas An organ of the digestive system located behind the stomach.

Pap test (Pap smear) Examination of a sample of cells collected from the cervix and the vagina.

passive smoking (secondhand smoke) Exposure to other people's tobacco smoke. This is a risk factor for lung cancer.

pelvic exam A vaginal and rectal examination by the doctor of the vagina, vulva, cervix, fallopian tubes, and ovaries.

pelvis The lower part of the abdomen located between the hip bones. Organs in a woman's pelvis are the uterus, vagina, ovaries, fallopian tubes, bladder, and rectum.

percutaneous needle biopsy A procedure in which a sample of lung tissue is obtained by a needle inserted through the skin.

pernicious anemia A blood disorder caused by a lack of vitamin B_{12}. People with this disorder do not produce the substance in the stomach that allows the body to absorb vitamin B_{12}. This condition is a risk factor for stomach cancer.

pesticide A chemical used for killing insects or fungi.

Philadelphia chromosome (Ph[1]) An abnormality of chromosome 22 that is seen in bone marrow and blood cells of most patients with chronic myelogenous leukemia and some with acute lymphocytic leukemia.

picocurie (pCi) A unit of measurement of radioactivity. It is one trillionth of a curie. Radon is typically measured in picocuries per liter.

polyp A mass of tissue that develops on the inside wall of a hollow organ. Polyps may become cancerous and should be removed.

precancerous A condition that is not malignant, but may eventually become so.

primary prevention Ways to keep cancer from ever occurring.

progesterone A female hormone that is instrumental in preparing the uterus for pregnancy.

promotion An event that follows *initiation* to cause cancer.

radiation therapy (radiotherapy) Treatment with high-energy rays from X-rays or other sources to kill cancer cells.

radon   An invisible, naturally occurring, inert radioactive gas that comes from uranium. It can cause lung cancer.

rectum   The last six to eight inches of the large intestine.

relative risk   Comparison of the incidence of a particular cancer among people with a specific risk factor with its incidence among people without the risk factor.

relative survival rate   A survival rate that takes normal life expectancy into account; the likelihood that a patient will not die of his or her disease by some specified time after diagnosis.

risk factor   A trait, habit, or characteristic that has been shown to be associated with increasing a person's chance of getting a particular disease.

RNA (ribonucleic acid)   A nucleic acid present in all living cells that controls protein synthesis by translating the genetic information within the cell.

screening   An examination for a disease, such as cancer, in a person or a specific population without symptoms.

secondary prevention   Detection of cancer as early as possible, so as to ensure the best chance of survival.

sidestream smoke   This is the smoke that goes directly into the air from the smoldering tobacco of a cigarette, pipe, or cigar. It accounts for most (90 percent) of the gasses and particles in environmental tobacco smoke indoors. It is a risk factor for lung cancer.

slab-on-grade construction   A term describing the construction of a house on a flat bed of concrete, generally without a basement or crawl space.

sonogram   see "ultrasonography."

spinal tap   A procedure in which a needle is used to withdraw fluid surrounding the spine for microscopic examination.

A spinal tap may be used in the diagnosis of brain cancer, breast cancer, leukemia, and other cancers.

sputum   A mucous secretion from the lungs that is expelled through the mouth. Examination of the sputum for cancer cells may be used in the diagnosis of lung cancer.

squamous intraepithelial lesion (SIL)   A general term for the abnormal growth of squamous cells on the surface of the cervix. SIL can be high grade or low grade and is considered a precancerous condition.

staging   A system of classifying a disease's severity or extent in the body.

stomach   A muscular pouch that helps in the digestion of food by mixing it with digestive juices and churning it into a thin liquid.

stool   The solid waste discharged in a bowel movement. Blood found in the stool may be an indication of colorectal cancer.

tertiary prevention   Reducing a disease's rate of recurrence and disability.

thoracotomy   Surgery through the chest wall. This procedure may be performed in the diagnosis of lung cancer.

transvaginal ultrasonography (transvaginal sonography, TVS)   Use of an internal vaginal probe in combination with ultrasound for the detection of ovarian cancer.

tumor   An abnormal mass of tissue that can be benign or cancerous.

tumor marker   A substance in the blood or other body fluid that can suggest that a person has cancer. Tumor markers are also used to detect a recurrence of cancer.

tumor suppressor genes   Genes in the body that can stop or block the development of cancer.

ultrasonography   A test in which sound waves are bounced off tissues and the echoes are converted into a picture called a *sonogram.* Ultrasound can be used in the diagnosis of many cancers, including breast, pancreas, ovarian, uterine, and Hodgkin's disease.

upper GI (gastrointestinal) series   A series of X-rays of the esophagus, stomach, and small intestine that are taken after you drink a barium solution, a white, chalky substance that outlines the organs on the X-ray.

urethra   The tube leading from the bladder to the outside of the body.

urinalysis   A test that analyzes the content of urine.

uterus (womb)   In females, the small, pear-shaped, muscular organ in the pelvis where the embryo, then fetus can develop.

vagina   In females, the muscular canal extending from the cervix to the outside of the body.

X-ray   High-energy radiation, used in low doses to diagnose disease and in high doses to treat cancer.

ℒᴏ

Organizations and Resources

GENERAL

American Association of Retired Persons (AARP), 601 E Street NW, Washington, DC; (202) 434–2560; (800) 424–3410. Provides legislative advocacy for programs such as Medicare; provides insurance supplemental to Medicare.

American Brain Tumor Association (ABTA), 2720 River Road, Suite 146, Des Plaines, IL 60018; (800) 886–2282. Provides patient education publications, information about treatment facilities, and a triannual newsletter.

American Cancer Society (ACS), 1599 Clifton Road NE, Atlanta, GA; (404) 320–3333; the toll-free cancer response line is (800) ACS–2345 and is in operation from 8:30 A.M. to 4:30 P.M. ACS is a nationwide voluntary health organization. It supports and funds research; provides education on cancer prevention, early detection, and treatment; provides services for cancer patients and their families; and provides free literature. There are 57 chartered divisions and about 3,000 local units. The following are the chartered divisions by state:

Alabama: 505 Brookwood Blvd., Homewood, AL 35209; (205) 879–2242.

Alaska: 406 West Fireweed Lane, Anchorage, AK 99503; (907) 277–8696.

Arizona: 2929 East Thomas Road, Phoenix, AZ, 85016; (602) 224–0524.

Arkansas: 901 N. University, Little Rock, AR 72207; (501) 664–3480.

California: 1710 Webster Street, Oakland, CA 94612; (510) 893–7900.

Colorado: 2255 South Oneida, PO Box 24669, Denver, CO 80224; (303) 758–2030.

Connecticut: Barnes Park South, 14 Village Lane, Wallingford, CT 06492; (203) 265–7161.

Delaware: 92 Read's Way, New Castle, DE 19720; (302) 324–4227.

District of Columbia: 1875 Connecticut Ave., Washington, DC 20009; (202) 483–2600.

Florida: 3709 West Jetton Ave., Tampa, FL 33629–5146; (813) 253–0541.

Georgia: 2200 Lake Blvd., Atlanta, GA 30319; (404) 816–7800.

Hawaii: Community Services Center Bldg., 200 N. Vineyard Blvd., Honolulu, HI 96817; (808) 531–1662.

Idaho: 2676 Vista Ave., Boise, ID 83705–0836; (208) 343–4609.

Illinois: 77 E. Monroe, Chicago, IL 60603–5797; (312) 641–6150.

Indiana: 8730 Commerce Park Place, Indianapolis, IN 46268; (317) 872–4432.

Iowa: 8364 Hickman Road, Suite D, Des Moines, IA 50325; (515) 253–0147.

Kansas: 1315 S.W. Arrowhead Road, Topeka, KS 66604; (913) 273–4114.

Kentucky: 701 W. Muhammad Ali Blvd., Louisville, KY 40203–1909; (502) 584–6782.

Louisiana: Fidelity Homestead Bldg., 837 Gravier Street, Suite 700, New Orleans, LA 70112–1509; (504) 469-0021.

Maine: 52 Federal Street, Brunswick, ME 04011; (207) 729–2339.

Maryland: 8219 Town Center Drive, White Marsh, MD 21162–0082; (301) 931–6850.

Massachusetts: 30 Speen Street, Farmingham, MA 01701 (508) 720–4600.

Michigan: 1205 E. Saginaw Street, Lansing, MI 48906; (517) 371–2920.

Minnesota: 3316 W. 66th Street, Minneapolis, MN 55435; (612) 925–2772.

Mississippi: 1380 Livingston Lane, Lakeover Office Park, Jackson, MS 39213; (601) 362–8874.

Missouri: 3322 American Ave., Jefferson City, MO 65102; (314) 893–4800.

Montana: 313 N. 32nd Street, Suite #1, Billings, MT 59101; (406) 252–7111.

Nebraska: 8502 W. Center Road, Omaha, NE 68124-5255; (402) 393–5800.

Nevada: 1325 E. Harmon, Las Vegas, NV 89119; (702) 798–6857.

New Hampshire: 360 Route 101, Unit 501, Bedford, NH 03110–5032; (603) 472–8899.

New Jersey: 2600 Route 1, CN 2201, North Brunswick, NJ 08902; (908) 297–8000.

New Mexico: 5800 Lomas Blvd. NE, Albuquerque, NM 87110; (505) 260–2105.

New York: 6725 Lyons Street, PO Box 7, East Syracuse, NY 13057; (315) 437–7025.

• Long Island: 75 Davids Drive, Hauppauge, NY 11788; (516) 436–7070.

• New York City: 19 W 56th Street, New York, NY 10019; (212) 586–8700.

• Queens: 112–25 Queens Blvd., Forest Hills, NY 11375; (718) 263–2224.

• Westchester: 30 Glenn Street, White Plains, NY 10603; (914) 949–4800.

North Carolina: 11 S. Boylan Ave., Raleigh, NC 27603; (919) 834–8463.

North Dakota: 123 Roberts Street, PO Box 426, Fargo, ND 58107; (701) 232–1385.

Ohio: 5555 Frantz Road, Dublin, OH 43017; (614) 889–9565.

Oklahoma: 4323 63rd Street, Suite 110, Oklahoma City, OK 73116; (405) 843–9888.

Oregon: 0330 SW Curry, Portland, OR 97201; (503) 295–6422.

Pennsylvania: PO Box 897, Route 442 & Sipe Ave., Hershey, PA 17033–0897; (717) 533–6144.

• Philadelphia: 1626 Locust Street, Philadelphia, PA 19103; (215) 985–5400.

Puerto Rico: Calle Alverio #577, Esquina Sargento Medina, Hato Rey, PR 00918; (809) 764–2295.

Rhode Island: 400 Main Street, Pawtucket, RI 02860; (401) 722–8480.

South Carolina: 128 Stonemark Lane, Columbia, SC 29210; (803) 750–1693.

South Dakota: 4101 Carnegie Place, Sioux Falls, SD 57106–2322; (605) 361–8277.

Tennessee: 1315 Eighth Ave. South, Nashville, TN 37203; (615) 255–1227.

Texas: 2433 Ridgepoint Drive, Austin, TX 78754; (512) 928–2262.

Utah: 941 East 3300 S, Salt Lake City, UT 84106; (801) 483–1500.

Vermont: 13 Loomis Street, PO Box 1452, Montpelier, VT 05601–1452; (802) 223–2348.

Virginia: PO Box 6359, Glen Allen, VA 23058–6359; (804) 527–3700.

Washington: 2120 First Ave. North, Seattle, WA 98109–1140; (206) 283–1152.

West Virginia: 2428 Kanawha Blvd. East, Charleston, WV 25311; (304) 344–3611.

Wisconsin: PO Box 902, Pewaukee, WI 53072–0902; (414) 523–5500.

Wyoming: 2222 House Ave., Cheyenne, WY 82001 (307) 638–3331.

American College of Radiology, 1891 Preston White Drive. Reston, VA 22091. (800) 227–5463.

American Lung Association, 1740 Broadway, New York, NY 10019; (212) 315–8700. Local chapters offer information on smoking cessation classes, self-help support groups, and video stop-smoking programs free on loan. Check your phone book for your local chapter or contact the national organization.

American Medical Association (AMA), 515 North State Street, Chicago, IL 60610; (312) 464–5000.

Board Certification, (800) 776–2378. Can provide information on whether a doctor is board certified. (The *Directory of Medical Specialists* lists the qualifications of medical doctors and should be available in medical libraries and the public library.)

Cancer Care, 1180 Ave. of the Americas, New York, NY 10036; (212) 221–3300. A nonprofit social service agency; helps patients and family members cope with the emotional and financial consequences of cancer; it generally serves the New York metropolitan area but responds to phone calls and letters from all over the United States, providing information and referrals whenever possible.

Cancer Information Service (CIS), a nationwide toll-free service, (800) 4–CANCER or (800) 422–6237. Funded largely by the National Cancer Institute. Cancer information specialists can tell callers the latest state-of-the-art treatment for a particular cancer, where clinical trials are taking place, as well as provide information about detection, prevention, diagnosis, support groups, and FDA certified mammography facilities; free NCI booklets are available.

Centers for Disease Control and Prevention (CDC), Office of Public Affairs, 1600 Clifton Road NE, Atlanta, GA 30333 (404) 329-3286. Answers public's questions on health-related issues.

Hereditary Cancer Institute, Henry Lynch, M.D., Creighton University School of Medicine, California at 24th, Omaha, NB 68178; (402) 280–2942. Provides free cancer-risk information and other forms of genetic counseling.

International Bottled Water Association (IBWA), (800) 928–3711. Represents 85 percent of bottled-water manufacturers; can give you information on bottled water from a particular company.

International Myeloma Foundation, 2120 Stanley Hills Drive, Los Angeles, CA 90046; (800) 452–CURE. Has a newsletter and provides information.

Leukemia Society of America, 600 Third Ave., New York, NY 10016. (800) 955–4LSA. Has 57 local chapters; provides information on leukemia, lymphomas, and multiple myeloma; may provide financial assistance for outpatient chemotherapy drugs and therapy, transportation, and transfusions.

Make Today Count, 1235 East Cherokee, Springfield, MO 65804–2263; (800) 432–2273. Provides support groups, brochures, and handouts for people with cancer and other life-threatening illnesses.

National Black Leadership Initiative on Cancer (NBLIC), Executive Plaza North, Room 240-D, Bethesda, MD 20892. (301) 496–8589; fax (301) 496–8675. A community-based outreach program specifically targeting African-Americans; it is a program of the NCI.

National Cancer Institute, NIH Building 31, Room 10A18, Bethesda, MD 20892; (301) 496–5583. The cancer arm of the National Institutes of Health; provides research, training, and information on all aspects of cancer prevention, detection, and treatment; operates the Cancer Information Service.

National Coalition for Cancer Survivorship (NCCS), 1010 Wayne Ave., 5th Floor, Silver Spring, MD 20910; (301) 650–8868. A network of independent groups and individuals offering support to cancer survivors, family members, and friends; provides information and resources on support and life after a cancer diagnosis, with special attention to job and insurance discrimination; advocates for rights of survivors.

National Hispanic Leadership Initiative on Cancer, South Texas Health Research Center, University of Texas Health Sciences Center at San Antonio, 7703 Floyd Curl Drive, San Antonio, TX 78284–7791; (210) 614–4496; fax (210) 615–0661. A community based outreach program targeting the Hispanic population.

National Women's Health Network, 1325 G Street NW, Washington, DC 20005; (202) 347–1140. Advocacy organization for women's health.

Office of Alternative Medicine, OAM/NIH, 6120 Executive Blvd., Suite 450, Rockville, MD 20892–9904; (301) 402–2466; fax (301) 402–4741. Has various fact sheets on alternative treatments; part of the National Institutes of Health.

Older Women's League (OWL), PO Box 1242, Ansonia Station, New York, NY 10023–1409.

Skin Cancer Foundation, 245 Fifth Ave., Suite 2402, New York, NY 10016; (212) 725–5176. Supplies education, information, pamphlets, and services related to skin cancer.

U.S. Food and Drug Administration (FDA), 5600 Fishers Lane, Rockville, MD 20857; (800) 332–1088; (301) 443–4190. A government agency that provides information on federal regulation of drugs.

ASBESTOS

TSCA Assistance Information Service (EPA) Asbestos Hotline, 401 M Street SW, Washington, DC 20460; (202) 554–1404. Provides information and publications on regulations under the Toxic Substances Control Act and the EPA's asbestos programs; free publications.

Regional Asbestos Coordinators from the U.S. Environmental Protection Agency: Region 1 (Connecticut, Maine, Massachusetts, New Hampshire, Rhode Island, Vermont): Regional Asbestos Coordinator, USEPA, JFK Federal Building, Boston, MA 02203; (617) 565–3836.

Region 2 (New Jersey, New York, Puerto Rico, Virgin Islands): Regional Asbestos Coordinator, USEPA, 2890 Woodbridge Ave., Edison, NJ 08837; (201) 321–6671.

Region 3 (Delaware, District of Columbia, Maryland, Pennsylvania, Virginia, West Virginia): Regional Asbestos Coordinator, USEPA, 841 Chestnut Bldg., Philadelphia, PA 19107; (215) 597–3160.

Region 4 (Alabama, Florida, Georgia, Kentucky, Mississippi, North Carolina, South Carolina, Tennessee): Regional Asbestos Coordinator, USEPA, 345 Courtland Street NE, Atlanta, GA 30365; (404) 347–3059.

Region 5 (Illinois, Indiana, Michigan, Minnesota, Ohio, Wisconsin): Regional Asbestos Coordinator, USEPA, 77 West Jackson Blvd., Chicago, IL 60604; (312) 886–6003.

Region 6 (Arkansas, Louisiana, New Mexico, Oklahoma, Texas): Regional Asbestos Coordinator, USEPA, 1445 Ross Ave., Dallas, TX 75202; (214) 665–7581.

Region 7 (Iowa, Kansas, Missouri, Nebraska): Regional Asbestos Coordinator, USEPA, 726 Minnesota Ave., Kansas City, KS 66101; (913) 551–7391.

Region 8 (Colorado, Montana, North Dakota, South Dakota, Utah, Wyoming): Regional Asbestos Coordinator, USEPA, 999–18th Street, Suite 500, Denver, CO 80295; (303) 293–1442.

Region 9 (Arizona, California, Guam, Hawaii, Nevada): Regional Asbestos Coordinator, USEPA, 75 Hawthorne Street, San Francisco, CA 94105; (415) 744–1128.

Region 10 (Alaska, Idaho, Oregon, Washington): Regional Asbestos Coordinator, USEPA, 1200 Sixth Ave., Seattle, WA 98101; (206) 553–0110.

BREAST CANCER

Breast Implant Information Network, (800) 887–6828. Provides assistance and information to women with implants or who are considering getting them; material packets and newsletters are available.

National Alliance of Breast Cancer Organizations (NABCO), 9 East 37th Street, 10th floor, New York, NY 10016; (212) 889–0606. An advocate for breast cancer patients and survivors. NABCO has a newsletter. It prefers inquiries be sent.

National Breast Cancer Coalition (NBCC), 1707 L Street NW, Suite 1060, Washington, DC 20036; (202) 296–7477; fax (202) 265–6854; national advocacy group for breast cancer.

National Lymphedema Network (NLN), 2211 Post Street, Suite 404, San Francisco, CA 94115; (800) 541–3259; fax (415) 921–4284. The hot line provides emotional support, educational information, and referrals to health-care professionals, treatment centers, local support groups, and exercise programs.

Susan G. Komen Breast Cancer Foundation, 3005 LBJ Freeway, Suite 370, Dallas, TX 75244; (214) 980–8841; (800) I'M AWARE or (800) 462–9273. Funds breast cancer research, education, screening, and treatment; has publications available; sponsors "Race for the Cure"; has toll-free hot line.

U.S. Food and Drug Administration (FDA), 5600 Fishers Lane, Rockville, MD 20857; (301) 245–8012; (800) 532–4400. Provides information on breast implants and mammography.

Y-ME, 18220 Harwood Ave., Homewood, IL 60430; (708) 799–8338; fax (708) 799–8228; hot line (800) 221–2141. Offers information, advocacy, and support; has a prosthesis and wig bank for women with financial need.

DIET/NUTRITION

American Dietetic Association, (800) 366–1655. Has recorded messages and publications; you can also speak with a dietician.

Center for Food Safety and Applied Nutrition, U.S. Food and Drug Administration, 200 C Street SW, Room 3321, Washington, DC 20204; (202) 245–1236. Provides information on nutrition, food, food technology, and food additives.

Center for Science in the Public Interest, 1501 16th Street NW, Washington, DC 20036; (202) 332–9110. Dedicated to improving the American diet through research, education, and advisory services.

New York-Cornell Medical Center in New York, operates a garlic hot line at (800) 330–5922.

Public Voice for Food and Health Policy, 1001 Connecticut Ave. NW, Suite 522, Washington, DC 20036. Acts as a national consumer "watchdog" organization; monitors food and health agencies and congressional committees charged with protecting public health.

Soy Protein Council, 1255 23rd Street NW, Suite 850, Washington, DC 20037; (202) 467–6610. Provides information on research and government actions.

United Soybean Hotline, (800) TALK SOY. For recipes and information.

U.S. Department of Agriculture (USDA), Center for Nutrition Policy and Promotion, 1120 20th Street, Suite 200, North Lobby, Washington, DC 20036; (202) 418–2312; fax (202) 208–2321. Makes available many free publications on dietary guidelines, food preparation, shopping for foods, bag lunches, snacks and desserts, and more.

U.S. Food and Drug Administration (FDA), Consumer Inquiries, 5600 Fishers Lane, Rockville, MD 20857; (301) 443–3170. Answers questions and supplies publications related to food and drug safety and efficacy.

ENVIRONMENTAL

Greenpeace, 1017 W. Jackson, Chicago, IL 60607; (312) 666–3305. Organization investigating the role of various environmental hazards in the development of cancer.

Indoor Air Quality Information Clearinghouse (IAQ/INFO), PO Box 37133, Washington, DC 20013–7133; (800) 438–4318; (202) 484–1307; fax (202) 484–1510. This service of the EPA offers free publications on toxins in the home or workplace.

National Institute of Environmental Health Services (NIEHS), 100 Capitol Drive, Suite 108, Durham, NC 27713; (800) 643–4794; fax (919) 361–9408. Sponsors ENVIRO-HEALTH Clearinghouse; free publications.

U.S. Environmental Protection Agency (EPA), 4001 M Street, Washington, DC 20460; (202) 829–3535. Provides information on hazards in the environment.

Women's Environmental and Development Organization (WEDO), 845 Third Ave., 15th floor, New York, NY 10022; (212) 759–7892. Has newsletter and does advocacy on issues involving women and the environment.

PESTICIDES

American Chemical Society, 1155 16th Street NW, Washington, DC 20013; (202) 872–4515.

Center for Science in the Public Interest, 1875 Connecticut Ave., NW, Suite 300, Washington, DC 20009; (202) 332–9110. Advocacy organization, has publications on environmental issues.

Concern, Inc., 1794 Columbia Road NW, Suite 6, Washington, DC 20009; (202) 238–8160. Advocacy organization for environmental issues.

Council for Agricultural Science and Technology (CAST), 137 Lynn Ave., Ames, IA 50010–7197; (515) 292–2125. Publishes reports on alternative agriculture and the relationship between pesticides and cancer.

Hazardous Materials Information Hotline, Center for Hazardous Materials Research, University of Pittsburgh Applied Research, 320 William Pitt Way, Pittsburgh, PA 15238; (800) 334–2467. Provides information on pesticides, hazardous waste, waste reduction, and recycling.

Household Products Disposal Council, 1201 Connecticut Ave. NW, Suite 300, Washington, DC 20036; (202) 659–5535. Provides information on the proper disposal of hazardous household wastes, such as cleaning agents, pesticides, and household disinfectants.

National Coalition Against the Misuse of Pesticides (NCAMP), 701 E Street SE, Suite 200, Washington, DC 20003; (202) 543–5450. Information on research, health effects and alternatives; advocacy group.

National Coalition for Alternatives to Pesticides (NCAP), PO Box 1393, Eugene, OR 97440; (503) 344–5044. Information on nontoxic ways to eliminate hazards presented by pests and fungi.

Natural Resources Defense Council, 71 Stevenson Street, Suite 1825, San Francisco, CA 94105; (415) 777–0220.

Pesticide Action Network, North American Regional Center, 965 Mission Street, Suite 514, San Francisco, CA 94103; (415) 541–9140.

Public Citizen, 215 Pennsylvania Ave., Washington, DC 20003; (202) 546–4994. Has publications on pesticides, radon; research and advocacy group.

Rachel Carson Council, 8940 Jones Mill Road, Chevy Chase, MD 20815; (301) 652–1877. Has free publications and will help people having difficulties with pesticides.

U.S. Environmental Protection Agency (EPA), (202) 382–2902. National Pesticides Telecommunications Network (under the EPA) (800) 858–7378. In operation weekdays 6:30 A.M.–4:30 P.M. Pacific time for information on pesticides.

RADON

State Government Radon Contacts:

Alabama (800) 582–1856

Alaska (800) 478–4845

Arizona (800) 225–4845

Arkansas (501) 661–2301

California (800) 745–7236

Colorado (800) 846–3986

Connecticut (203) 566–3122

Delaware (800) 554–4636

District of Columbia (202)
   727–5728

Florida (800) 543–8279

Georgia (800) 745–0037

Hawaii (808) 586–4700

Idaho (800) 445–8647

Illinois (800) 325–1245

Indiana (800) 272–9723

Iowa (800) 383–5992

Kansas (913) 296–1560

Kentucky (502) 564–3700

Louisiana (800) 256–2494

Maine (800) 232–0842

Maryland (800) 872–3666

Massachusetts (413) 586–7525

Michigan (517) 335–8190

Minnesota (800) 798–9050

Mississippi (800) 626–7739

Missouri (800) 669–7236

Montana (406) 444–3671

Nebraska (800) 334–9491

Nevada (702) 687–9354

New Hampshire (800) 852–3345
   ext. 4674

New Jersey (800) 648–0394

New Mexico (505) 827–4300

New York (800) 458–1158

North Carolina (919) 571–4141
North Dakota (701) 221–5188
Ohio (800) 523–4439
Oklahoma (405) 271–5221
Oregon (503) 731–4014
Pennsylvania (800) 237–2366
Puerto Rico (809) 767–3563
Rhode Island (401) 277–2438
South Carolina (800) 768–0362
South Dakota (605) 773–3351
Tennessee (800) 232–1139
Texas (512) 834–6688
Utah (801) 538–6734
Vermont (800) 560–0601
Virginia (800) 468–0138
Washington (800) 323–9727
West Virginia (800) 922–1255
Wisconsin (608) 267–4795
Wyoming (800) 458–5847

SMOKING

Action on Smoking and Health (ASH), 2013 H Street NW, Washington, DC 20006; (202) 659–4310. Nonprofit smoking group; provides general information.

American Cancer Society, 1559 Clifton Road NE, Atlanta, GA 30329; (800) ACS–2345. Has materials on smoking and runs "Fresh Start" smoking cessation classes; see "General" section for local offices.

Americans for Nonsmokers' Rights, 2530 San Pabli Ave., Suite J, Berkeley, CA 94702; (510) 841–3032. Advocacy organization.

American Lung Association, 1740 Broadway, New York, NY 10019–4374; (212) 315–8700. Provides help for smokers who want to quit through their Freedom From Smoking self-help smoking cessation program; actively supports legislation and information campaigns for nonsmokers' rights.

Indoor Air Quality Information Clearinghouse (IAQ/INFO), PO Box 37133, Washington, DC 20013–7133; (800) 438–4318; (202) 484–1307; fax (202) 484–1510. This service of the EPA offers free publications on the hazards of cigarette smoking.

National Cancer Institute's Cancer Information Service, (800) 4–CANCER. Has free publications on smoking and can make referrals to smoking cessation programs.

National Heart, Lung, and Blood Institute, Information Center, PO Box 30105, Bethesda, MD 20824–0105. Has information on smoking.

National Institute for Occupational Safety and Health, 4676 Columbia Parkway, Cincinnati, OH 42226–1998; (800) 35–NIOSH.

Office on Smoking and Health, Centers for Disease Control and Prevention, Mail Stop K-50, 4770 Buford Highway NE, Atlanta, GA 30341–3724; (800) CDC–1311. Answers questions, makes referrals, and publishes a bulletin related to smoking and health.

WORKPLACE

U.S. Department of Labor, Occupational Safety and Health Administration (OSHA), Directorate of Technical Support, 200 Constitution Ave. NW, Washington, DC 20210; (202) 219–7047. Can provide information regarding work-related hazards and occupational injuries and illnesses.

Comprehensive Cancer Centers

(DESIGNATED BY THE NATIONAL CANCER INSTITUTE
AS OF 1996)

ALABAMA
University of Alabama Comprehensive Cancer Center, 1918 University Blvd., Basic Health Sciences Bldg., Room 108, Birmingham, AL; (205) 934–5077.

ARIZONA
University of Arizona Cancer Center, 1501 North Campbell Ave., Tucson, AZ 85724; (602) 626–6372.

CALIFORNIA
Jonsson Comprehensive Cancer Center, University of California at Los Angeles, 100 UCLA Medical Plaza, Suite 255, Los Angeles, CA 90027; (213) 206–0278.

The Kenneth Norris Jr. Comprehensive Cancer Center, University of Southern California, 1441 Eastlake Ave., Los Angeles, CA 90033–0804; (213) 226–2370.

CONNECTICUT
Yale University Comprehensive Cancer Center, 333 Cedar Street, New Haven, CT 06510; (203) 785–4095.

DISTRICT OF COLUMBIA
Lombardi Cancer Research Center, Georgetown University Medical Center, 3800 Reservoir Road NW, Washington, DC 20007; (202) 687–2192.

FLORIDA
Sylvester Comprehensive Cancer Center, University of Miami Medical School, 1475 Northwest 12th Ave., Miami, FL 33136; (305) 545–1000.

MARYLAND
The Johns Hopkins Oncology Center, 600 North Wolfe Street, Baltimore, MD 21205; (301) 955–8964.

MASSACHUSETTS
Dana-Farber Cancer Institute, 44 Binney Street, Boston, MA 02115; (617) 632–3476.

MICHIGAN
Meyer L. Prentis Comprehensive Cancer Center of Metropolitan Detroit, 110 East Warren Avenue, Detroit, MI 48201; (313) 745–4329.

University of Michigan Cancer Center, 101 Simpson Drive, Ann Arbor, MI, 48109–0752; (313) 936–9583.

MINNESOTA
Mayo Comprehensive Cancer Center, 200 First Street Southwest, Rochester, MN 55905; (507) 284–3413.

NEW HAMPSHIRE
Norris Cotton Cancer Center, Dartmouth-Hitchcock Medical Center, 2 Maynard Street, Hanover, NH 03756; (603) 646–5505.

NEW YORK
Columbia Presbyterian Medical Center, Comprehensive Cancer Center, 630 West 168th Street, New York, NY 10032; (212) 305–9327.

Memorial Sloan-Kettering Cancer Center, 1275 York Ave., New York, NY 10021; (800) 525–2225.

Roswell Park Cancer Institute, Elm and Carlton Streets, Buffalo, NY 14263; (800) 761–9355.

NORTH CAROLINA

Cancer Center of Wake Forest University at the Bowman Gray School of Medicine, 300 South Hawthorne Road, Winston-Salem, NC 27103; (919) 748–4354.

Duke Comprehensive Cancer Center, PO Box 3814, Durham, NC 27710; (919) 684–2748.

Lineberger Comprehensive Cancer Center, University of North Carolina School of Medicine, Chapel Hill, NC 27599; (919) 966–4431.

OHIO

Ohio State University Comprehensive Cancer Center, 410 West 10th Ave., Columbus, OH 43210; (800) 638–6996.

PENNSYLVANIA

Fox Chase Cancer Center, 7701 Burholme Ave., Philadelphia, PA 19111; (215) 728–2570.

Pittsburgh Cancer Institute, 200 Meyran Ave., Pittsburgh, PA 15213–2592; (800) 537–4063.

University of Pennsylvania Cancer Center, 3400 Spruce Street, Philadelphia, PA 19104; (215) 662–6364.

TEXAS

The University of Texas M.D. Anderson Cancer Center, 1515 Holcombe Blvd., Houston, TX 77030; (713) 792–3245.

San Antonio Cancer Institute, 8122 Datapoint Drive, Suite 600, San Antonio, TX 78229; (210) 616-5590.

VERMONT

Vermont Cancer Center, University of Vermont, 1 South Prospect Street, Burlington, VT 05401; (802) 656–4580.

WASHINGTON

Fred Hutchinson Cancer Research Center, 1124 Columbia Street, Seattle, WA 98104; (206) 667–5000.

WISCONSIN

Wisconsin Clinical Cancer Center, University of Wisconsin, 600 Highland Ave., Madison, WI 53792; (608) 263–8090.

Bibliography

Altman, Roberta, and Michael Sarg, M.D. *The Cancer Dictionary*. New York: Facts on File, 1992.

Altman, Roberta. *The Complete Book of Home Environmental Hazards*. New York: Facts on File, 1990.

Altman, Roberta. *Waking Up, Fighting Back: The Politics of Breast Cancer*. New York: Little, Brown and Company, 1996.

Baron-Faust, Rita. *Breast Cancer: What Every Woman Should Know*. New York: Hearst Books, 1995.

Beverly, Cal, ed. *Book of Proven Home Remedies and Natural Healing Secrets*. Peachtree City: FC and A Publishing, 1993.

Boston Women's Health Book Collective. *The New Our Bodies Ourselves: A Book by and for Women*. New York: Simon and Schuster, 1992.

Brady, Judy, ed. *1 in 3 Women with Cancer Confront an Epidemic*. Pittsburgh: Cleis Press, 1991.

Bruning, Nancy. *Breast Implants: Everything You Need to Know*. Alameda, CA: Hunter House Inc., 1995.

Cooper, Gary L., ed. *Stress and Breast Cancer*. New York: John Wiley and Sons, 1988.

Costello, Cynthia, and Anne J. Stone, eds. *The American Woman 1994–95: Where We Stand*. New York: W. W. Norton and Co., 1994.

Editors of the University of California at Berkeley *Wellness Letter*. *The Wellness Encyclopedia: The Comprehensive Family Resource for Safeguarding Health and Preventing Illness*. Boston: Houghton Mifflin Co., 1991.

Fink, John M. *Third Opinion: An International Directory to Alternative Therapy Centers for the Treatment and Prevention of Cancer*

and Other Degenerative Diseases. Garden City Park, NY: Avery
Publishing Co., 1988.

Gershoff, Ph.D., and Catherine Whitney. *The Tufts University Guide
to Total Nutrition.* New York: Harper and Row, 1990.

Johnson, Judi, and Linda Klein. *I Can Cope: Staying Healthy with
Cancer.* Wayzata, MN: DCI Publishing, 1994.

Kemeny, M. Margaret, M.D., and Paula Dranov. *Breast Cancer &
Ovarian Cancer: Beating the Odds.* Reading: Addison-Wesley
Publishing Company Inc., 1992.

Komarnicky, Lydia, M.D., and Anne Rosenberg, M.D., with Marian
Betancourt. *What To Do If You Get Breast Cancer.* Boston: Little,
Brown and Co., 1995.

Laurence, Leslie, and Beth Weinhouse. *Outrageous Practices: The
Alarming Truth About How Medicine Mistreats Women.* New York:
Ballantine Books, 1994.

Love, Susan M., M.D., with Karen Lindsey. *Dr. Susan Love's Breast
Book,* 2nd ed. Reading: Addison-Wesley Publishing Co. Inc.,
1995.

Margen, Sheldon, M.D., and the editors of the University of California at Berkeley *Wellness Letter. The Wellness Encyclopedia of
Food and Nutrition.* New York: Rebus, 1992.

Morra, Marion, and Eve Potts. *Choices.* New York: Avon Books,
1994.

Moss, Ralph W., Ph.D. *Cancer Therapy: The Independent Consumers Guide to Nontoxic Treatment and Prevention.* New York: Equi-
nox Press, 1992.

Moss. *The Cancer Industry: The Classic Exposé on the Cancer Establishment.* New York: Paragon House, 1991.

Murphy, Gerald, Walter Lawrence, Jr., and Raymond Lenhard, Jr.,
eds. *American Cancer Society Textbook of Clinical Oncology.* Atlanta: American Cancer Society, 1995.

Nechas, Eileen, and Denise Foley. *Unequal Treatment: What You
Don't Know About How Women are Mistreated by the Medical
Community.* New York: Simon and Schuster, 1994.

Northrup, Christiane, M.D. *Women's Bodies, Women's Wisdom: Cre-
ating Physical and Emotional Health and Healing.* New York: Ban-
tam Books, 1994.

Office of Technology Assessment. *Unconventional Cancer Treatments.* Washington, DC: U.S. Government Printing Office, 1990.

The PDR Guide to Women's Health and Prescription Drugs. Montvale, NJ: Medical Economics, 1994.

Prevention Magazine Health Books Editors. *The Complete Book of Cancer Prevention.* Emmaus, PA: Rodale Press, 1988.

Somer, Elizabeth, M.A., R.D. *Nutrition for Women, The Complete Guide.* New York: Henry Holt and Co., 1993.

Walters, Richard. *Options: The Alternative Cancer Therapy Book.* Honesdale, PA: Paragon Press, 1993.

Winawer, Sidney J., M.D., and Moshe Shike, M.D. *Cancer Free, The Comprehensive Prevention Program.* New York: Simon and Schuster, 1995.

Index

abortion, breast cancer and, 11
Adamson, Richard, 33
adenomas, 113
adenosis, sclerosing, 25–26
adrenal glands, 55
aerosols, 11–12
age
    cancer risk and, 12, 55–56
    mammography and, 89–90
    of menarche, 55, 189
    of oral contraceptive use, 101
    at pregnancy, 56, 114
air pollution
    hazardous wastes and, 195
    indoor, 157
    industrial, 183–84
    secondhand smoke, 4, 176–78
alar, 107–08
alcohol consumption, 13–14, 50, 54, 83,
    94
aldrin, 198
allium compounds, 111
allylic sulfides, 74, 111
American Cancer Association, 28
American Cancer Institute, 13, 132
American Cancer Society, 34, 39, 51, 76,
    89, 134
American College of Sports Medicine
    (ACSM), 58
American Institute for Cancer Research,
    13
American Medical Women's Association,
    83
American Physical Society, 193
analgesics, with phenacetin, 185
Anderson, David E., 80
ankylosing spondylitis, 123
antioxidants, 14–15, 21–22, 126, 148
arsenic and arsenic compounds, 185
artificial sweeteners, 15–17

asbestos
    eliminating, 160–62
    in home, 159–62
    organizations and resources, 237–38
aspartame, 16, 17
aspirin, 17–18
azathioprine, 185

bacillus thuringiensis (Bt), 200
barbecued foods, 19–20, 40–41
Beatson, George Thomas, 55
benzene, 185–86
benzidine, 186
Bernstein, Leslie, 57–58
beta-carotene, 15, 21–22, 31
birth control pills. See Oral contracep-
    tives
bis-chloromethyl ether, 186
bladder cancer, 205
    anticancer drugs in, 187
    artificial sweeteners in, 15–17
    chlorinated water in, 151
    cigarette smoking in, 131
    coffee in, 40
    environmental chemicals in, 186, 187
bleeding
    between periods, 19, 54
    rectal, 87
block-wall ventilation method of radon
    reduction, 174
Blondell, Jerome, 164
bovine somatotropin (BST), 91–92
bowel
    contraction of, 57
    inflammatory disease, 87–88
    polyps in, 31
bowel cancer, 77
brain cancer, 33, 78
BRCA1 gene, 22–23
breads and grains
    calcium in, 32

253

fiber in, 66, 67
flaxseed in, 70
phytochemicals in, 111
vitamin A in, 143
vitamin C in, 145
vitamin E in, 148
breast
atypical hyperplasia of, 18, 26
lumps, 24–26
silicone implants, 128–29
breast cancer, 206
abortion in, 11
advocacy groups, 7
alcohol consumption in, 13, 50
bovine somatotropin (BST) in, 92
cigarette smoking in, 131, 132
coffee in, 40
electromagnetic fields in, 192–93
environmental chemicals in, 189–91
estrogen and, 11, 35, 43, 55–56, 84–85, 90, 96, 189
fat intake and, 60–61
gene for, 22–23
heredity in, 78, 80
hormone replacement therapy in, 84–85
lack of knowledge about, 1–2
among lesbians, 82–83
male, 3
menopause and, 90–91
obesity in, 58, 96
occupational hazards in, 178, 179
oral contraceptives in, 100–02
organizations and resources, 238–39
pesticides in, 36, 45, 46–47, 165, 188–89, 191–92, 198
supportive-expressive group therapy for, 121–22
vitamin A (retinoids) and, 142
x-rays in, 153
breast cancer prevention
breast-feeding and, 23–24
diet and, 21, 43–44, 66, 70, 75, 98, 110, 112, 126
exercise and, 57–58
pregnancy and, 113–15
prophylactic mastectomy and, 115–18
tamoxifen and, 37, 138–39
Breast Cancer Prevention Trial (BCPT), 37, 138–39
breast cancer screening
clinical exam, 39–40, 124–25
mammography, 3, 25, 26, 88–90, 125
self-exam (BSE), 27–31, 124–25
breast-feeding, breast cancer and, 23–24
broccoli, 31, 110, 111
bronchitis, chronic, 39
Burnett, Carol, 178

caffeic acid, 111
calcium
as chemoprevention agent, 38
deficiency, 42
food sources of, 31–32
in vegetables, 140–41
Calle, Eugenia, 132
cancer centers, by state, 245–48
carbon filtration, 152
Carson, Rachel, 183
Carter, Jimmy, 194
cauterization, 34
cellular phones, brain cancer and, 33
Centers for Disease Control and Prevention (CDC), 57, 58, 100–01, 178, 190, 191
cervical cancer, 206–07
antioxidants and, 15, 21
cigarette smoking in, 87, 131, 132
DES in, 48
human papillomavirus in, 86–87, 132
oral contraceptives in, 102
screening for, 34, 105–06, 125
sexual activity in, 87, 127–28
cervical dysplasia, 33–34, 70, 142
cervix, carcinoma in situ in, 70
Chassin, Mark, 190
cheese
calcium in, 32
low-fat, 62
nitrates and nitrites in, 95
chemicals
dioxin, 51
disinfectants, 165
dry cleaning, 52–53
in environment, 184–92
estrogenic, 35–36, 44–45, 46, 188–89
food additives, 95
in hazardous waste sites, 194–96
phytochemicals, 110–12, 135
in water supply, 151
See also drugs; pesticides
chemoprevention, 37–38
chlorambucil, 186
chlordane, 198
chlorine, in water, 150–51
chloromethyl methyl ether, 186
cholesterol-lowering drugs, 38–39
chromium and chromium compounds, 186
chronic obstructive pulmonary disease (COPD), 39
cigarette smoking, 83, 87
alcohol combined with, 14
as benzene source, 186
breast cancer and, 132
in cancer death rate, 131
cancers related to, 131–32

cervical cancer and, 87, 131, 132
lung cancer and, 4–5, 81, 131
oral cancer and, 54, 131
organizations and resources, 243–44
secondhand smoke, 4, 176–78
tips for quitting, 132–35
cleaning products, nontoxic, 165
clomiphene, 64, 65
coffee, 40, 47
Cohen, Kelman, 115, 116
colon cancer. *See* colorectal cancer
colorectal cancer, 207–08
alcohol consumption in, 13–14
Crohn's disease in, 42
fat intake in, 60, 61
heredity in, 77, 78, 79–80
inflammatory bowel disease in, 87–88
obesity in, 58, 97
polyps and, 31, 59, 73–74, 79–80, 113
screening for, 51, 97, 125, 128
colorectal cancer prevention
aspirin and, 17–18
chemoprevention agents and, 38
diet and, 21, 49, 66, 70, 98
exercise and, 57
Consumer Product Safety Commission, 159, 186
Coogan, Patricia, 192–93
copper
food sources of, 42, 140–41
protective effects of, 41–42
Crohn's disease, 42
cryosurgery, 34
cyclamates, 15–16
cyclophosphamide, 187
cysts, breast, 25

D & C (dilation and curettage), 54
dacthal (DCPA), 197
D'Argo, Joan, 188
DDT (dichloro-diphenyl-trichloroethane), 44–47, 165, 188–89, 191–92, 198
debrisoquine, 81
decaffeinated coffee, 47
depressurization, house, 174–75
DES (diethylstilbestrol), 48, 118, 125
diagnosis, early, 5
dicofol, 46
dieldrin, 198
diet
artificial sweeteners in, 15–17
beta-carotene in, 21–22
calcium in, 31–32, 44
coffee in, 40, 47
copper in, 42
fat intake and, 60–61, 64
fiber in, 31, 44, 49, 66–69, 72–73, 140–41

flaxseed in, 69–70
folic acid in, 70–71, 140–41
garlic in, 74
guidelines for, 49–50
iron in, 44
low-fat, 62–63
olive oil in, 98
omega-3 foods in, 99–100
organizations and resources, 239
phytochemical foods in, 31, 43, 110–12, 135
research on, 48–49
selenium in, 126–27
soybeans and soybean products in, 110, 112, 135–36
tea (green) in, 75–76
vitamin A in, 72–73, 140–41, 143–44
vitamin C in, 72–73, 140–41, 145–47
vitamin E in, 72–73, 140–41, 148–49
See also food preparation; *specific foods*
digital rectal exam, 51, 107, 125
dioxin, 51, 194
disinfectants, 165
dithiolthiones, 111
diuretics, 52
drain-tile suction method of radon reduction, 173–74
Dr. Susan Love's Breast Book, 30
drugs
anticancer, 186, 187, 201
anti-estrogen (tamoxifen), 37, 138–39
chemoprevention agents, 37
cholesterol-lowering, 38–39
fertility, 64–65
dry cleaning solvent, 52–53
dysplastic nevi, 93

electromagnetic fields (EMFs), 163, 179, 192–93
ellagic acid, 111
emphysema, 39
endometrial cancer, 215–16
hormone replacement therapy in, 85
hypertension in, 87
obesity in, 96
precancerous condition and, 53
endometrial hyperplasia, 53–54
endosulfan, 45–46, 198
environmental hazards, 183–204
environmental organizations, 240
Environmental Protection Agency (EPA), 107, 108, 150, 164, 165, 167, 170–71, 176, 183–84, 188, 194, 195, 197
Environmental Response, Compensation, and Liability Act (CERCLA), 195
Environmental Working Group, 46, 150

epigallocatechin gallate (EGCG), 75
Epstein, Samuel, 92, 138–39, 188
erythroplakia, 54
esophageal cancer
    alcohol consumption in, 14, 50
    cigarette smoking in, 131
    diet and, 3, 21, 75
    folic acid deficiency in, 70
    vitamin A and, 38
Estabrook, Alison, 45
estrogen
    anti-estrogen drugs, 138–39
    body fat and, 96
    breast cancer and, 11, 35, 43, 55–56,
        84–85, 90, 96, 189
    chemicals acting like, 34–36, 44–45,
        46, 188–89, 197–98
    conjugated, 186–87
    lifetime exposure to, 189
    replacement therapy, 84–86
ethylene dibromide (EDB), 108
exercise, 56–59

Falck, Frank, Jr., 45
familial adenomatous polyposis (FAP),
    59, 79–80
familial atypical multiple mole melanoma
    (FAMMM) syndrome, 60
fat, body, 96
fat, dietary
    cancer risk and, 60–61
    low-fat foods, 62–63
    recommended intake, 49, 64
    See also oils
fat necrosis, 25
fecal occult blood test, 97
Federal Insecticide, Fungicide, and Ro-
        denticide Act (FIFRA), 164–65
fenretinide, 142
fertility drugs, ovarian cancer and, 64–65
ferulic acid, 111
fiber, dietary
    benefits of, 66
    food sources of, 31, 44, 66–69
    in fruit, 72–73
    recommended intake, 49, 69
    in vegetables, 140–41
fibroadenoma, 25
fibrocystic disease, 24
fish
    low-fat, 20, 63
    nitrates and nitrites in, 95
    nutrients in, 32, 144, 147, 149
fish oil, 98–100
flaxseed, 69–70
folic acid
    deficiency, 42, 70

food sources of, 70–71
    in fruit, 72–73
    in vegetables, 31, 140–41
food
    nitrates and nitrites in, 95
    pesticides in, 45–46, 107–10
    See also diet; *specific foods*
Food and Drug Administration (FDA),
    15–17, 48, 76, 89, 92, 102, 108, 129,
    151
food preparation
    barbecuing, 19–20
    carcinogenic chemicals in, 40–41
    tips for, 71
formaldehyde, 165
4-aminobiphenyl, 185
free radicals, 14–15, 148
Freon, 12
fruit
    beta-carotene in, 21
    fiber in, 68–69
    nutrient chart, 72–73
    pesticides on, 108–09
    phytochemicals in, 110–11
    vitamin A in, 72–73, 143
    vitamin C in, 72–73, 145–46
    vitamin E in, 72–73, 149
Fugh-Berman, Adrian, 138

Galen, 119–20
Gardner's syndrome, 73–74, 80
garlic, 74, 111, 112
genetic counseling, 81, 118, 119
genistein, 110–11
genital warts. *See* human papillomavi-
        ruses
Goldberg, Itzhak, 189–90
Goldrich, Sibyl, 129
grains. *See* breads and grains
Grant, Ulysses, 120
granulated activated carbon (GAC) tank,
    152
Groth, Edward III, 53

hair dye, 76–77, 179
Haynes, Suzanne G., 82
hazardous wastes, 194–96
health insurance, 3
Healy, Bernadine, 138
heart disease, 84, 85
heat recovery ventilation (HRV), 172
Heier, Al, 107
Henrich, Janet, 84
hereditary nonpolyposis colorectal can-
        cer (HNPCC), 77
heredity, 60, 77, 78–81
heterocyclic aromatic amines (HAAs), 41

Hippocrates, 150
Hodgkin's disease, 123
Holland, Jimmie, 120
home, health hazards in, 157–78
homosexuality, breast cancer and, 82–83
Hooker Chemical Company, 194
hormone replacement therapy (HRT),
    84–86
Hughes, C.H., 120
human chorionic gonadotropin (HCG),
    64
human papillomaviruses (HPVs), 86–87,
    132
hyperplasia
    of breast, atypical, 18, 26
    endometrial, 53–54
    uterine, atypical, 19
hypertension, 87
hysterectomy, 125

immune system, 121
indole-3-carbinol, 43, 112
indoles, 111
insulinlike growth factor (IGF-1), 92–93
International Agency for Research on
    Cancer, 179
iron, food sources of, 44
isoflavones, 112, 135
isothiocyanates, 111

Jarrett, John R., 116–17

Kahn, Mary Jo, 117
kidney cancer, 208–09
    cigarette smoking in, 131
    diuretics in, 52
    obesity in, 58, 97
Klausner, Richard, 22

larynx cancer, 14, 38, 131
laser surgery, 34
lawn and garden care
    pesticides in, 197–98
    without pesticides, 198–200
legumes, 32
lesbians, breast cancer among, 82–83
LeShan, Lawrence, 120
leukemia, 209–10
    anticancer drugs in, 186, 187, 201
    benzene in, 186
    cigarette smoking in, 131
    electromagnetic fields in, 192
    hair dyes in, 78, 179
    heredity in, 76
    radiation in, 123, 153, 201
lignans, 69–70
limonene, 111

Lippman, Marc, 117
liver cancer, 50, 75, 185
Long Island, breast cancer rate in,
    189–91
Long Island Breast Cancer Study Project
    (LIBCSP), 190–91
Love, Richard, 138
Love, Susan, 30, 89, 118
Love Canal, 194
Lung Association, 134
lung cancer, 210–11
    asbestos exposure in, 159
    chronic obstructive pulmonary disease
        (COPD) in, 39
    cigarette smoking in, 4–5, 81, 131–32
    diet and, 21, 75
    environmental chemicals in, 185, 186
    gene for, 104
    heredity in, 78, 81
    incidence in women, 131
    radon exposure in, 167, 168
    secondhand smoke in, 176–77
    vitamin A and, 38, 123
Lynch syndromes, 77

MacMahon, Brian, 55
mammography, 3, 25, 26, 88–90
marinades, 20
mastectomy, prophylactic, 115–18
meat
    barbecued, 20
    cooking methods and, 40–41
    dioxin in, 51
    fat intake and, 61, 62–63
    folic acid in, 70
    nitrates and nitrites in, 95
    vitamin A in, 144
    vitamin C in, 147
    vitamin E in, 149
melanoma, 211
    heredity in, 60, 78, 80
    mole changes and, 93–94
    See also skin cancer
melphalan, 187
menopause
    age at, 56, 91
    breast cancer risk and, 90–91
    early (oophorectomy), 90
    hormone replacement therapy in, 84,
        85
menstruation
    age of menarche, 55, 189
    exercise and, 57
    heavy bleeding in, 19, 54
    ovulation, 103–04
methoxsalen with ultraviolet A (PUVA)
    therapy, 187

methoxychlor, 46, 198
milk
  bovine somatotropin (BST) in, 91–93
  calcium in, 31
  low-fat, 62, 91, 92
  soy, 135, 136
  vitamin A in, 144
mind-body connection, 120
miso, 136
moles, 93–94
mouth. *See* oral cancer
mouthwash, alcohol content of, 94
mustard gas, 187
myeloma, multiple, 76, 179

National Academy of Sciences, 107
National Cancer Institute (NCI), 3, 22,
  33, 37, 39, 46–47, 48–49, 66, 74, 75,
  81, 82, 89, 90, 94, 101, 134, 139,
  167, 190, 191, 195, 198
National Institute of Environmental
  Health Sciences (NIEHS), 190
National Institute of Occupational Safety
  and Health, 178
National Toxicology Program, 185
natural killer (NK) cells, 57
nitrates and nitrites, 95
nitrosamines, 95
non-Hodgkin's lymphoma, 76, 179, 185,
  198, 212
nonyl phenol, 35
Northrup, Christiane, 30
Norton, Larry, 61, 89, 90
nose cancer, 38, 131
nutrition. *See* diet; *specific nutrients*
nuts and seeds, 149

obesity, 3, 49, 58, 83, 96–97
Obrams, Iris, 191
occult blood stool test, 97, 125
occupational hazards, 178–79
Occupational Safety and Health Administration (OSHA), 196, 244
Office of Technology Assessment, 163
O'Hanlan, Katherine A., 82
O'Hara, John, 92
oils
  fish, 98–100
  olive, 98
Older Women's League (OWL), 3
Oldfield's syndrome, 80
olive oil, 98
omega-3 fatty acid, 98–100
1, 4-butanediol dimethanesulfonate, 186
onion, 74, 111, 112

oophorectomy
  breast cancer and, 90
  prophylactic, 119
oral cancer
  alcohol consumption in, 14, 50, 94
  beta-carotene and, 21
  cigarette smoking in, 54, 131
  erythroplakia in, 54
  vitamin A and, 38
oral contraceptives
  in breast cancer, 100–02
  protective effect of, 102–03
  in uterine cancer, 102
osteoporosis, 84, 85, 138
osteosarcoma, 105
ovarian cancer, 212–13
  diet and, 98
  exercise and, 57
  fat intake in, 60, 61
  fertility drugs in, 64–65
  hair dye in, 77
  heredity in, 78
  Lynch syndrome in, 77
  obesity in, 58, 96, 97
  oral contraceptives and, 103
  prophylactic oophorectomy and, 119
  talcum powder in, 137
ovarian hyperstimulation syndrome
  (OHSS), 65
ovaries, 55, 90
ovulation, 103–04
ozone layer depletion, 12
Ozonoff, David, 184

Paget, James, 120
Paget's disease, 105
pancreatic cancer, 213–14
  cigarette smoking in, 131
  coffee in, 40
  diet and, 75
  Lynch syndrome in, 77
papilloma, intraductal, 26
Pap test, 34, 48, 87, 105–06, 125
PBBs, 191
Pearson, Cindy, 27
pelvic cancer, 131
pelvic exam, 107, 125
perchloroethylene, 52–53
pest control, nontoxic, 165, 200
pesticides
  arsenic in, 185
  breast cancer and, 36, 45, 46–47, 188–
    89, 191–92, 198
  in environment, 196–97
  estrogenic, 35–36, 44–45, 46, 188–89,
    197–98
  on foods, 45–46, 107–10

hazardous wastes, 194
  in home, 164–67
  on lawn and garden, 197–200
  limiting exposure to, 36–37, 47, 108–
    10, 165–67
  organizations and resources, 240–41
  regulation of, 164–65
  water contamination and, 151
p53 gene, 104
pharynx cancer, 14, 38, 94, 131
phenacetin, in analgesics, 185
phenethyl isothiocyanate (PEITC), 110
Physicians Health Study, 17
phytic acid, 111
Phytochemicals, 31, 43, 110–12, 135
phytosterols, 112
Pike, Malcolm, 115
plastics, estrogenlike chemicals in, 35
polychlorinated biphenyls (PCBs), 194
polynuclear aromatic hydrocarbons
    (PAH), 41
polyps, colorectal, 31, 59, 73–74, 113
Postmenopausal Estrogen/Progestin In-
    terventions (PEPI) Trial, 85
Pozniak, Marie, 194
pregnancy
  age at first, 56, 114
  breast cancer and, 113–15
  delayed, 178
pressurization, house, 175
progesterone and progestin, 85
prophylactic surgery, 81
  mastectomy, 115–18
  oophorectomy, 119
prostate cancer, 61, 70
protease inhibitors, 112
protein, soy, 135, 136
psychological factors, 119–22

radiation
  cancer rate and, 201
  limiting exposure to, 153–54, 202
  therapy, 123
  x-rays, 152–54
radon
  EPA guidelines, 170–71
  in home, 167–76
  reduction methods, 171–76
  state government contacts, 242–43
  testing for, 169–70
  in water, 151, 152, 168
rectal cancer. *See* colorectal cancer
rectal exam, digital, 51, 107, 125
Reichman, Marsha E., 13
Resource Conservation and Recovery
    Act (RCRA), 195
retinoids, 123, 141–42, 144

risk factors
  categories of, 2–3, 6
  combinations of, 4
  gender and, 3
Roentgen, Wilhelm, 152–53
Rogers, Adrianne, 142
Roosevelt, Theodore, 16
Rose, David, 64

saccharin, 16
saponins, 112
screening
  for cervical cancer, 34, 105–06, 125
  for colorectal cancer, 51, 97, 125, 128
  for skin cancer, 126, 130–31, 203–04
  See also breast cancer screening; *spe-
    cific tests*
secondhand smoke, 4, 176–78
selenium, 38, 126–27
Seligman, Paul, 178
Senie, Ruby, 36
sexual behavior, 87, 127–28
Shittemore, Alice, 64
Shumway, John, 91
sigmoidoscopy, 125, 128
Silent Spring (Carson), 183
Silent Spring Institute, 46
silicone breast implants, 128–29
skin cancer, 214
  antioxidants and, 15
  chemoprevention agents and, 37, 38
  diet and, 75
  environmental chemicals in, 185
  screening for, 126, 130–31, 203–04
  sun exposure in, 2, 12, 202–04
  vitamin A and, 123
  See also melanoma
smoking. *See* cigarette smoking
Sondik, Ed, 82
Sonnenschein, Carlos, 35
Soto, Anna, 35, 46
soybeans and soybean products, 110,
    112, 135–36
Spicer, Darcy, 102
Spiegel, David, 121–22
squamous intraepithelial lesion (SIL).
    See cervical dysplasia
stomach cancer, 215
  cigarette smoking in, 131
  diet and, 21, 43, 75
  folic acid deficiency in, 70
  Lynch syndrome in, 77
stool
  fiber intake and, 66
  test, occult blood, 97
stress. *See* psychological factors

sub-slab suction method of radon reduction, 174
sugar, 50
sugar substitutes, 15–17
sulforaphane, 31, 43
sun, exposure to, 2, 12, 202–04
supportive-expressive group therapy, 121–22
Surgeon General's report, on smoking, 131

Talalay, Paul, 110
talcum powder, ovarian cancer and, 137
tamoxifen, 37, 138–39
tea, green, 75–76
tempeh, 135
Theriault, Richard, 55
throat cancer, 50
tofu, 135
Tomato, 110
total trihalomethanes (TTHMs), 150–51, 152
toxaphene, 198
Toxic Substances Control Act (TSCA), 195
trichlorethylene (TCE), 47
Trichopoulos, Dimitri, 114
Turcot's syndrome, 80
2, 4-D, 198
2-naphthylamine, 187
2-toluene diamine (TDA), 129

ulcerative colitis, 87–88
ultrasound, 25
U.S. Department of Agriculture, 13, 50
uterine cancer, 215–16
  atypical uterine hyperplasia in, 19
  beta-carotene and, 21
  diet and, 98
  dioxin in, 51
  exercise and, 57
  Lynch syndrome in, 77
  obesity in, 58, 96
  oral contraceptives and, 102–03
  tamoxifen in, 139
uterine hyperplasia, atypical, 19

vaginal cancer, DES and, 48
vegetables
  beta-carotene in, 21–22
  calcium in, 32
  cruciferous, 31, 43–44, 111
  fiber in, 68
  folic acid in, 70–71
  grilled, 20
  nutrient chart, 139–41

pesticides on, 45–46, 108–09
phytochemicals in, 110–12
vitamin A in, 140–41, 143–44
vitamin C in, 140–41, 146–47
vitamin E in, 140–41, 148
ventilation, for radon reduction, 171–72
vinyl chloride, 187–88
vitamin A, 15, 21, 31
  as chemoprevention agent, 37–38
  in fruit, 72–73, 143
  in grain products, 143
  in meat, 144
  in milk, 144
  retinoids, 123, 141–42, 144
  in vegetables, 140–41, 143–44
vitamin B_{12}, 42
vitamin C
  as chemoprevention agent, 38
  copper absorption and, 42
  in fruit, 72–73, 145–46
  in grains, 145
  in meat, 147
  supplements, 144–45
  in vegetables, 31, 140–41, 146–47
vitamin E
  in fruit, 72–73, 149
  in grains, 148
  in meats, 149
  in nuts and seeds, 149
  selenium and, 126
  in vegetables, 140–41, 148
vitamins and minerals
  as chemoprevention agents, 37–38
  deficiencies in, 42
  See also specific nutrient

Warthin, Alfred Scott, 78
water
  arsenic in, 185
  chlorinated, 150–51
  contaminated, 150, 151–52, 168, 195, 197
Watras, Stanley, 168
weight control, exercise and, 58
Welsch, Clifford, 142
Whall, Clifford, 94
Wolff, Mary S., 36, 190
Women's Bodies, Women's Wisdom (Northrup), 30
Women's Health Network, 102, 138
workplace, health hazards in, 178–79, 244

x-rays, diagnostic, 152–54

Yang, Chung S., 75